Catheter Ablation of Persistent Atrial Fibrillation: A Practical Guide

REMEDICA ✳

Published by Remedica

Commonwealth House, 1 New Oxford Street, London, WC1A 1NU, UK
Civic Opera Building, 20 North Wacker Drive, Suite 1642, Chicago, IL 60606, USA
Tel: +44 20 7759 2999
Fax: +44 20 7759 2901
Email: books@remedica.com
www.remedica.com

Publisher: Andrew Ward
In-house editors: Catherine Booth, James Griffin, Leonard Wills
Design and artwork: AS&K Skylight Creative Services

© 2008 Remedica

Remedica is a member of the AS&K Media Partnership.

ISBN-13: 978-1-905721-49-8

British Library Cataloguing-in-Publication Data
A catalogue record for this book is available from the British Library.

Printed in Malta

Catheter Ablation of Persistent Atrial Fibrillation: A Practical Guide

Mark O'Neill, George Veenhuyzen, and Sébastien Knecht

Mark O'Neill, MB BCh BAO DPhil
Department of Cardiology
St Mary's Hospital
London, UK

George Veenhuyzen, MD
Libin Cardiovascular Institute of Alberta
and University of Calgary
Foothills Hospital
Calgary, Alberta
Canada

Sébastien Knecht, MD
Service de Rythmologie
Hôpital Cardiologique du Haut-Lévêque
Bordeaux, Pessac
France

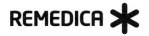

Table of contents

Preface

Over the course of the last decade, there has been an exponential rise in the number of catheter ablation procedures performed for atrial fibrillation (AF). Electrical confirmation of pulmonary vein isolation is now widely accepted as the endpoint for the treatment of patients with paroxysmal AF, and cure rates in excess of 80% are not uncommon in centers achieving this endpoint. The successful treatment of persistent AF continues to present a daunting challenge to the interventional cardiac electrophysiologist, not least because of the absence of such a clear procedural endpoint. Despite very welcome advances in catheter location and electrogram analysis technologies, there remains little in the way of consensus as to the best approach to the treatment of this pernicious arrhythmia.

Over the last 5 years, our group has developed a systematic and reproducible approach to the treatment of persistent AF, which aims to restore sinus rhythm by ablation alone. In so doing, we have learned an appreciation for the fascinating electrophysiology that underpins this arrhythmia. This book is an attempt to integrate, in a practical fashion, an ablation technique that works with the electrophysiology behind it. Furthermore, we try to show how this can be achieved with the relatively simple electrophysiological equipment available in electrophysiology laboratories already performing more conventional ablation procedures.

The book has been deliberately written more in the style of a manual than as a reference text, although we hope that it may serve as both. It is divided according to how we see the phases of an ablation procedure for persistent AF: pulmonary vein isolation, electrogram-guided ablation, and linear ablation. Accurate mapping of atrial tachycardia is critical to the successful restoration of sinus rhythm in these patients, and also in dealing with the consequences of catheter ablation therapy: clinical arrhythmia recurrences, which in the majority of patients are in the form of atrial tachycardias, including macro re-entrant, localized re-entry, or true focal point tachycardias. Finally, the book follows a real clinical case from start to finish in an effort to illustrate how a systematic and sequential approach to treatment, using the AF cycle length as a marker of procedural progress, can lead to, dare we say, cure of an arrhythmia previously believed to be incurable.

The book is intended as a starting point for individuals motivated by a desire to understand the electrophysiological mechanisms at work in this chaotic arrhythmia. The approach detailed herein dissects these mechanisms as revealed by the ablation technique described, and is heavily illustrated in a way in which we hope can be understood by all true students of electrophysiology, among whom we count ourselves.

Mark O'Neill, MB BCh BAO DPhil
George Veenhuyzen, MD
Sébastien Knecht, MD

Acknowledgments

We are indebted to Michel Haïssaguerre, Pierre Jaïs, and Mélèze Hocini for their support and encouragement throughout the preparation of this book. We acknowledge the important contributions of current and recent generations of staff, fellows, and visitors to pass through the atrial fibrillation service at the Hôpital Cardiologique in Bordeaux, France including Seiichiro Matsuo, Kang-Teng Lim, Leonardo Arantes, Sathish Kodali, Nicolas Derval, Frédéric Sacher, Yoshi Takahashi, Anders Jönsson, Prashanthan Sanders, Antoine Deplagne, Julien Laborderie, Mats Jensen-Urstad, and, in particular, George Klein. Finally, we are extremely grateful to our wives, Marianne, Shazia, and Jan, for giving us the time and freedom to compile this book together, despite our geographical separation.

Forewords

Atrial fibrillation (AF) has become the number one indication for interventional catheter ablation in large volume centers around the world.

The publication of *Catheter Ablation of Persistent Atrial Fibrillation: A Practical Guide* is a welcome addition to the literature on the approach to investigating catheter ablation of AF. During its writing, I had the pleasure of hosting Dr George Klein in our laboratory, which stimulated numerous discussions and encouraged an atmosphere of learning.

This practical manual, authored by Dr Mark O'Neill, Dr George Veenhuyzen, and Dr Sébastien Knecht, describes what we see on a daily basis when huddled around a bright monitor in a darkened laboratory. The authors have harvested many electrograms during a number of AF ablation procedures. They describe a pragmatic approach to the targeting of such electrograms and provide what we believe to be the mechanism underlying specific activation patterns. This interpretation is confirmed in most cases by successful local ablation, as defined by a change in AF cycle length and/or termination of AF.

Despite the unprecedented success of this approach to catheter ablation of chronic AF – and several examples are shown in this manual where the technique restores sinus rhythm – we are fully aware of our ignorance in interpreting signals during chaotic activation with multiple areas of fractionated activity. Currently, we have only rudimentary mapping tools to help identify the individual elements involved in AF, but there is still a long way to go before we fully understand and master this arrhythmia.

In order to facilitate learning, all sections are supported by images, which will be invaluable both to the electrophysiologist and the technician. If this manual encourages readers to further investigate electrogram interpretation in AF, and fosters their curiosity in deciphering the language of the electrogram, then a major goal of this book has been achieved.

Michel Haïssaguerre, MD

Hôpital Cardiologique du Haut-Lévêque
and the Université Victor Segalen Bordeaux II
Bordeaux, France

It has been difficult not to observe the focus, energy, and passion of the 'Bordeaux' group in pursuing a practical, evidenced-based ablative cure of atrial fibrillation (AF) for more than a decade. The landmark observation of rapid firing in and around the pulmonary veins, and the description of pulmonary vein isolation, turned the tide and provided the basis for truly effective ablative procedures. A flood of manuscripts from Bordeaux subsequently documented the evolution of their progress, describing novel mechanistic insights in addition to practical and technical expediencies. As well as paroxysmal AF in the relatively normal heart, the group has described a systematic method for dealing with the still challenging frontier of long-standing AF and that associated with heart failure. The 'sequential' approach is an acknowledgment of complex, eclectic, and highly individual mechanisms in patients with persistent AF. The procedure provides a disciplined approach in the face of overwhelming complexity where the mechanisms driving AF are cryptic but gradually overcome as the procedure progresses. Although complex technologies have been used in Bordeaux, it is noteworthy that these outstanding achievements have been made largely with relatively fundamental tools and a fallback to 'classical' electrophysiological principles, patience, and emphasis on good technique.

Drs O'Neill, Veenhuyzen, and Knecht have done a superb job of bringing together the crux of this information in one volume. They have provided us with a detailed and well-illustrated manual of the 'Bordeaux' technique and the philosophy as it stands today, which students of this discipline will find indispensable.

George J. Klein, MD

Division of Cardiology
University of Western Ontario
London, Ontario, Canada

1 | Introduction: rationale, practical aspects, and equipment

This chapter describes the equipment and techniques used in our laboratory for ablation of chronic atrial fibrillation. Particular emphasis is placed on the importance of the atrial fibrillation cycle length in guiding the procedure and informing our understanding of the arrhythmia itself.

- Rationale

- Practical aspects

- Equipment

- Signal processing

- Atrial fibrillation cycle length

- Measuring the atrial fibrillation cycle length

- Left atrial nomenclature

Rationale

The use of catheter ablation to isolate the pulmonary veins (PVs) has proven effective in the majority of patients with paroxysmal atrial fibrillation (AF), but largely ineffective in patients with persistent AF, underscoring the importance of other structures in the maintenance of the fibrillatory process. Persistent AF is a complex arrhythmia that represents the sum of multiple profibrillatory elements, all of which need to be considered for ablation in an individual patient in order to restore sinus rhythm. From an anatomic perspective the PVs, inferior left atrium (LA) and coronary sinus (CS), left atrial appendage (LAA), and septum are consistent sites at which ablation has an impact on fibrillation, as determined by prolongation of the atrial fibrillation cycle length (AFCL) measured in the LAA and right atrial appendage (RAA). The multiple electrophysiological mechanisms at work in driving AF are gradually revealed by increasing left and right atrial ablation, and include localized re-entry, focal-point activity, and macro re-entry. Our approach to catheter ablation of persistent AF is based upon recognition of these electrophysiological mechanisms within their anatomic context, thereby permitting ablation targeting the triggering and perpetuating mechanisms of AF.

As the procedure progresses, AF is gradually converted from a chaotic process to one that is slower and more organized, and therefore amenable to mapping. Once the anatomic or electrophysiological substrate maintaining AF ceases to be present (typically when the AFCL reaches 180–200 ms or longer in the presence of amiodarone), AF terminates by conversion to either atrial tachycardia (AT) or sinus rhythm. There are often multiple different ATs occurring in the context of the ablated atrium, where intra- and interatrial conduction properties may be severely deranged, thereby adding significant complexity to the procedure. These tachycardias constitute the last, but frequently the most difficult, step in ablation for persistent AF. However, mapping and ablation of these has become an indispensable step in the process of AF ablation and is the difference between procedural success and failure.

Practical aspects

The approach outlined in this book currently leads to the termination of AF in 85% of cases, without the need for intraprocedural pharmacologic or electrical cardioversion (ie, by ablation alone). After a mean of 1.6 procedures/patient, sinus rhythm is maintained in 95% of patients after a follow-up of 2 years.

Patients with symptomatic persistent AF who are refractory to antiarrhythmic drug therapy are candidates for the procedure if they accept the benefits and risks, including a >50% chance of requiring a second procedure. Patients are not excluded on the basis of LA size, duration of AF, or the presence of concomitant structural heart disease. After an initial procedure where AF is terminated by catheter ablation alone, only 5% of patients will experience recurrent AF. Interestingly, when AF cannot be terminated during the first procedure (and the patient is electrically cardioverted), 40% of patients will experience recurrent AF. This underscores the importance of AF termination as a procedural endpoint.

In persistent AF of less than 5 years' duration, the baseline AFCL is the most important predictor of AF termination by ablation. An AFCL of <140 ms at the outset is associated with a longer procedure and a lower likelihood of restoring sinus rhythm. The AFCL is measured at "sentinel" sites (ie, the LAA and RAA) and is closely correlated with the AFCL estimated from lead V1, meaning that an electrocardiogram (ECG) can be used as a simple tool to predict the amount of ablation that might be required.

Therapeutic anticoagulation with warfarin is required for at least 1 month prior to the procedure. A transesophageal echocardiogram (TEE) is performed within 48 hours prior to the procedure to exclude the possibility of an LA thrombus, which is present in approximately 1% of cases despite anticoagulation. Warfarin is discontinued 48 hours prior to ablation and substituted with low-molecular-weight heparin (LMWH) up to and including the morning of the procedure. All antiarrhythmic drugs are stopped for at least five half-lives prior to ablation with the exception of amiodarone, which is continued.

Following ablation, antiarrhythmic medication may be continued for up to 3 months at the operator's discretion, and warfarin continued for at least 6 months, after which the decision to continue warfarin is made based on the individual patient's thrombotic risk profile. Patient follow-up is performed with Holter monitoring at 1, 3, and 6 months, and at 6-monthly intervals thereafter. Longer duration follow-up with closed loop or implantable technologies will provide more precise information on long-term outcome.

Equipment

Sedation is achieved with midazolam and morphine, and additional anesthetist-administered sufentanil as required. Three sheaths are placed in the right common femoral vein, and a steerable catheter is placed in the CS such that its tip is at the 3 o'clock position in the 30° left anterior oblique (LAO) view. Transseptal puncture is performed with pressure monitoring and contrast injection through the transseptal needle to confirm LA access prior to advancing the dilator and sheath assembly. A guidewire is advanced to a left PV and the dilator and sheath are pulled back into the right atrium (RA) to allow passage of an externally irrigated ablation catheter with a 3.5 mm distal electrode (THERMOCOOL; Biosense Webster, Inc, Diamond Bar, CA, USA) through the puncture site. The dilator and sheath are then advanced over the guidewire into the LA alongside the ablation catheter. Here, they are aspirated, and flushed initially and then continuously with heparinized dextrose at 100 mL/hour. A bolus of heparin (50 U/kg) is administered immediately after LA access, and again after 4 hours for procedures lasting >4 hours. The activated clotting time is not routinely monitored.

Signal processing

During these procedures, 12-lead surface ECGs and bipolar endocardial ECGs are continuously monitored and stored using a digital amplifier and computer recording system (LabSystem PRO; Bard Electrophysiology, C R Bard, Inc, Lowell, MA, USA). All signals are sampled at 1 kHz, with filter settings from 30 to 250 Hz for intracardiac signals and from 0.1 to 50 Hz for surface ECGs.

Intracardiac signals are displayed at an amplification of 0.1 mV/cm and with a gain of 16× for the mapping catheter, and 0.2 mV/cm with 8× gain for the CS as well as the PENTARAY and LASSO catheters (Biosense Webster, Inc, Diamond Bar, CA, USA). The tracings provided in this book were obtained using these methods unless otherwise stated.

Atrial fibrillation cycle length

Computer-modeling studies have been used to validate the AFCL as a measure of the complexity of AF. The AFCL represents the population of elements contributing to the fibrillatory process; the greater the number of such elements, the more complex the AF and the shorter the AFCL. Furthermore, the minimum AFCL is dictated by the atrial refractory period, while the number of elements contributing to AF is theoretically very great. This may explain why ablation within the LA is not always accompanied by a change in AFCL. **Figure 1.1** demonstrates the hypothesis that: (a) the number of elements contributing to AF is related to the AFCL; and (b) as ablation removes individual elements, there is a nonuniform increase in AFCL, with some sites resulting in a greater increase than in others. The flat portion of the curve represents those elements where elimination has no impact on AFCL.

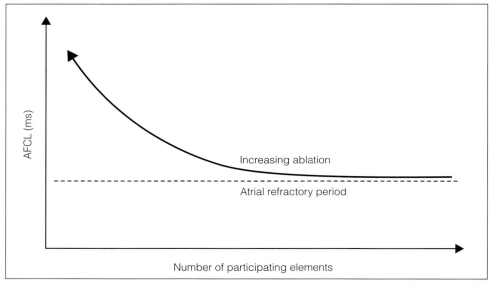

Figure 1.1. Atrial fibrillation cycle length (AFCL) and the number of participating elements.

Measuring the atrial fibrillation cycle length

Electrograms (EGMs) in persistent AF are complex and cannot be reliably evaluated in terms of cycle length (CL), except in both appendages. The steerable CS catheter can be placed in the RAA and the ablation catheter in the LAA to measure simultaneously the left and right AFCLs at the beginning of the procedure. Using custom analysis software (Bard Electrophysiology, C R Bard, Inc, Lowell, MA, USA), the mean AFCL for the selected window is calculated. The EGM annotation is then verified manually online to ensure accuracy (**Figure 1.2**). Inter-EGM intervals of <100 ms or continuous electrical activity are manually corrected to count as a single interval. However, the EGM within the LAA is always discrete and of high amplitude, thereby facilitating unambiguous automatic annotation of this EGM.

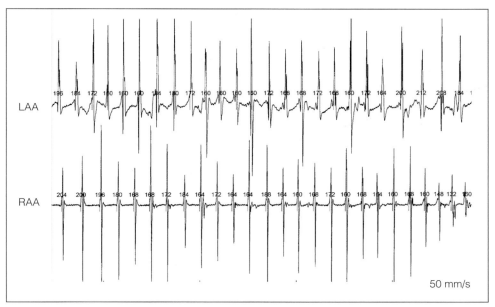

Figure 1.2. Automatic atrial fibrillation cycle length annotation from electrograms recorded in the left atrial appendage (LAA) and right atrial appendage (RAA).

In the absence of analysis software, the mean AFCL can be estimated by measuring the total duration required for 10 cycles (or longer) and dividing that number by 10 (or the number of cycles measured) (**Figure 1.3a**). Following PV isolation, the circumferential mapping catheter is placed within the RAA. A bipole displaying a discrete RAA EGM is selected and displayed in real time. The AFCL may then be assessed simultaneously over 10–30 cycles within the LAA and RAA throughout the procedure to follow the impact of ablation. The AFCL can often be reliably estimated from V1 on the 12-lead ECG in a patient with persistent AF (**Figure 1.3b**).

A 20-mm circular decapolar catheter (LASSO; **Figure 1.4a**) is advanced via the transseptal sheath (SL0; St Jude Medical, St Paul, MN, USA) and positioned just distal to the PV ostia to map the PV perimeter during pulmonary vein isolation (PVI). A multispine 20-pole catheter (PENTARAY; **Figure 1.4b**) can be used to map focal atrial activation during organized AF or nonmacro re-entrant tachycardias that arise after AF terminates. While not routinely required, various 3D electroanatomic mapping technologies may be used for the assessment of anatomy, EGM analysis, and quantification of the impact of ablation on LA and RA voltages. Occasionally, these technologies are useful for mapping ATs that may arise after AF termination or during subsequent procedures.

Radiofrequency energy (RF) is delivered using a Stockert generator (Biosense Webster, Inc, Diamond Bar, CA, USA) with the power settings shown in **Table 1.1**. These power settings have been determined empirically to provide effective lesions while minimizing the risks of PV stenosis, steam pops, cardiac tamponade, and collateral damage to the phrenic nerve, esophagus, and circumflex coronary artery. Target temperatures of 40–45°C are achieved (maximum temperature 50°C) by manual titration of irrigation rates from 5–60 mL/minute (0.9% saline via COOLFLOW pump; Biosense Webster, Inc, Diamond Bar, CA, USA).

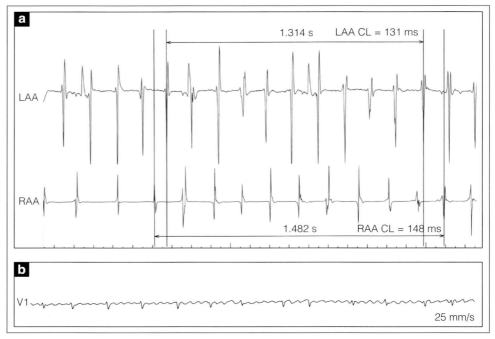

Figure 1.3. Manual atrial fibrillation cycle length (AFCL) annotation from electrograms recorded in the left atrial appendage (LAA) and right atrial appendage (RAA).

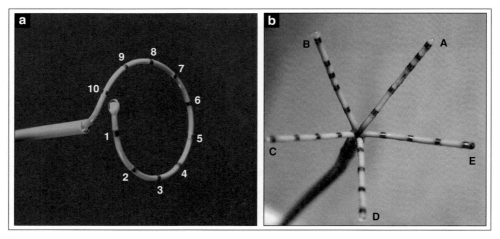

Figure 1.4. (a) The LASSO circular decapolar catheter; **(b)** the PENTARAY multispine catheter.

Once sinus rhythm has been restored, the integrity of PVI and linear ablation is verified and, if not already done, linear ablation of the cavotricuspid isthmus (CTI) is performed. Thus, the endpoints for the procedure include the restoration of sinus rhythm, PVI, and bidirectional conduction block at sites of linear ablation.

Site of ablation	Power (W)	Typical ablation time (mins)
PVs	25–30	25–35
LA roof	25–30	10–15
Posterior LA	25	3–6
Anterior LA	25–30	3–6
Inferior LA	30–35	5–10
LA septum	25–35	3–6
Coronary sinus	20–25	4–8
Right atrium	25–30	0–20
Mitral isthmus	30–35	10–20
Cavotricuspid isthmus	30–35	8–12

Table 1.1. Stockert generator power settings and typical ablation times for various ablation sites. LA: left atrium; LAA: left atrial appendage; PV: pulmonary vein.

After the procedure, patients receive LMWH injections, beginning on the evening of the day that ablation takes place and continuing until the international normalization ratio is in the therapeutic range. Warfarin is continued for at least 6 months, and thereafter its dosing is guided by the presence or absence of conventional risk factors for thromboembolism and the maintenance of sinus rhythm. All antiarrhythmic drugs are discontinued by 3 months, except in the case of arrhythmia recurrence. In this setting, patients are listed for a repeat procedure.

At 1, 3, 6, and 12 months, patients are admitted to hospital for 24 hours to undergo clinical evaluation, including exercise stress testing, ambulatory monitoring, and transthoracic echocardiography.

Left atrial nomenclature

For descriptive purposes, the LA is divided into eight segments (**Figure 1.5**): the PV (shown in blue), LAA (shown in purple), anterior LA, LA roof, septal LA, posterior LA, inferior LA, and lateral LA. Atrial tissue 0.5–1.0 cm from the PV ostia is included within the PV region. The posterior LA approximates a square, the corners of which are defined

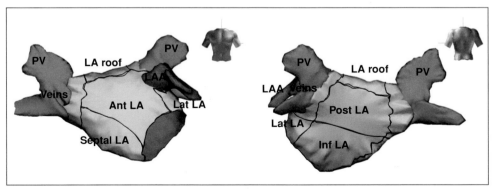

Figure 1.5. The eight segments of the left atrium (LA). Ant: anterior; Inf: inferior; Lat: lateral; LAA; left atrial appendage; Post: posterior; PV: pulmonary vein.

by the four PV orifices. The LA roof is arbitrarily defined as a band of 1–2 cm between the superior PVs, which separates the posterior LA from the anterior LA. The anterior LA extends from the LA roof to the superior mitral annulus (MA). The inferior LA extends from the lower aspect of the two inferior PV ostia to the inferior MA. The lateral LA is defined as atrial tissue between the posterolateral MA (at the 4 o'clock position) and the lower lip of the LAA. The septal LA extends from the right veins to the anteroseptal MA. Typical durations of RF delivery at each of these sites are given in **Table 1.1**.

2 | Pulmonary vein isolation

This chapter outlines the following aspects of pulmonary vein isolation and describes the interpretation of pulmonary vein electrograms in specific scenarios after catheter ablation.

- Pulmonary vein arrhythmogenic properties in sinus rhythm

- Pulmonary vein isolation techniques

- Pulmonary vein isolation during atrial fibrillation

- Left superior pulmonary vein isolation with atrial fibrillation confined inside the vein

- Right superior pulmonary vein isolation with atrial fibrillation confined inside the vein

Pulmonary vein arrhythmogenic properties in sinus rhythm

The identification of pulmonary vein (PV) ectopy is facilitated by the "dead end" configuration of PV muscular fascicles, resulting in opposing sequences of activation in ectopy versus sinus rhythm.

During sinus rhythm, near-synchronous potentials are recorded within the PV representing atrial and local PV activities (first complex). Once separated by ablation, pacing maneuvers, or spontaneous slow conduction, the first, low-amplitude potential represents activation of the adjacent left atrium (LA), or right atrium (RA) for the anterior part of the right PVs. It is usually synchronous with the first or second half of the P-wave for the right and left PVs, respectively.

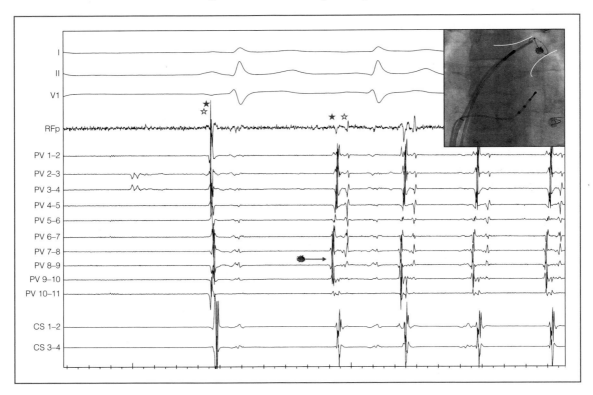

Figure 2.1. Pulmonary vein (PV) arrhythmogenic properties. The locally recorded atrial potentials are represented by open stars, and the locally recorded PV potentials by solid stars. CS: coronary sinus; p: proximal; RF: ablation catheter.

The second "sharp" potential reflects local activity from the PV striated musculature. When ectopy occurs in a PV (red spark, second complex) there is a reversal of the described activation sequence, with the pulmonary vein potential (PVP) preceding the LA potential (**Figure 2.1**).

Mapping of the earliest site of activity (arrow) during ectopy allows identification of discrete sites inside the vein, while the atrial exit site is dependent on the anatomy of the PV-LA connecting fascicles.

The inset radiograph depicts a circumferential mapping catheter in the left superior pulmonary vein (LSPV), an ablation catheter at the upper ostial aspect of the vein, and a quadripolar catheter in the coronary sinus (CS). The red spark depicts a schematic ectopic from the LSPV that propagates to the LA.

Pulmonary vein isolation techniques

Different eponyms have been used to describe PV isolation, but, in practice, there are more similarities than differences between these techniques. PVs can be isolated individually (**Figure 2.2a**) or as ipsilateral pairs ('*en bloc*') (**Figures 2.2b–d**) depending on venous anatomy, catheter stability, and the operator's preference. Whichever technique is selected, ablation should be performed 1–2 cm away from the PV ostia with a series of coalescent radiofrequency energy (RF) applications. However, a difference exists between the right and left PVs owing to the presence of the ridge separating the left atrial appendage (LAA) from the left PVs:

- Circumferential ablation can be performed around the right PVs with a continuous circular lesion.

- In contrast, ablation for the left PVs is usually started along the posterior wall (vertical line from high to low; **Figure 2.2b**) and followed by ablation within the first millimeters of the veins to target the fascicles lying anterior to the vein.

It is unusual to achieve PV isolation after circumferential coalescent lesions without further ablation targeting the earliest PV activity or sites of reverse PV polarity, as recorded on the circumferential mapping catheter indicating the residual anatomic connection.

Figures 2.2a and **b** are respective schematic representations of the ablation lesion set for individual and *en bloc* isolation of the left and right PVs. **Figure 2.2c** is a left anterior oblique (LAO) radiographic projection, upon which has been superimposed a computed tomography (CT) scan of the LA performed prior to the ablation procedure using custom Philips (Eindhoven, The Netherlands) CT overlay software. The CT image has been rendered transparent to facilitate visualization of the fluoroscopic anatomic landmarks, and the clipping plane allows visualization of the lesion set around the right PVs and along the septal posterior aspect of the left PVs. **Figure 2.2d** shows the complete opaque LA CT superimposed on the fluoroscopic image of the heart. The continuous anterior ablation lesions are clearly visible for the right PVs, while only two discrete lesions were needed on the anterior aspect of the LSPV to achieve isolation.

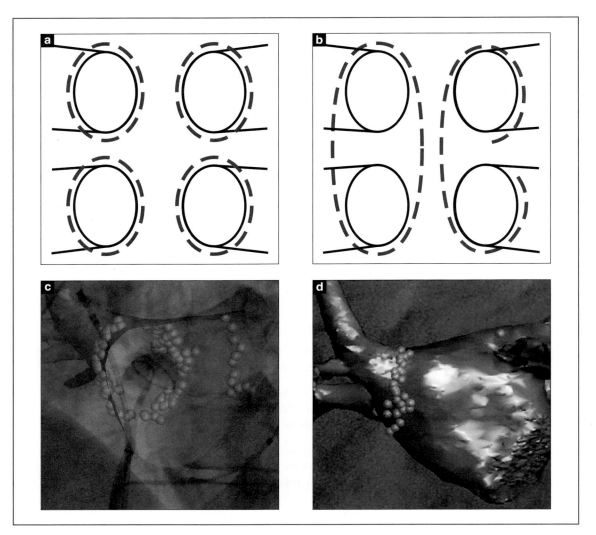

Figure 2.2. Pulmonary vein isolation techniques.

Pulmonary vein isolation during atrial fibrillation

During ongoing atrial fibrillation (AF), the sequence of PV activation is incessantly changing because: (a) multiple breakthroughs are present in most veins; (b) there are changing incident wave fronts of activation at the PV ostia; and (c) the LA-PV connections have rate-dependent conduction properties. A consistent activation sequence usually means discrete sites of breakthrough, either spontaneously or following prior ablation. Delivery of RF narrows the width or number of LA-PV connections, resulting in progressive consistency of the PV activation sequence.

In AF, far-field potentials can be distinguished from PV potentials using the following methods:

- The activation sequence of PV potentials is constantly changing during ablation, while that of far-field potentials is relatively stable.

- Consistent prolongation of PV cycle length (CL) may be observed due to a reduction of LA to PV connections with radiofrequency applications, helping to distinguish both potentials as illustrated in **Figure 2.3** (PV potentials are represented by stars).

- PV potentials represent local myocardial activation, and therefore exhibit sharper and larger tracings than those observed for the far-field potentials.

- If doubt remains, far-field potentials can be unmasked by putting a recording catheter in the suspected structure from which the far-field signal is emanating, eg, in the LAA. Synchronous activity between LAA and PV potentials confirms an external origin of potentials recorded on the circumferential catheter.

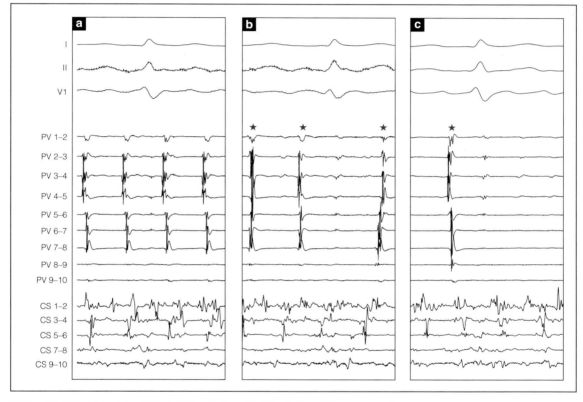

Figure 2.3. Pulmonary vein (PV) isolation during atrial fibrillation. CS: coronary sinus.

Figure 2.3 shows the recordings from three surface electrocardiogram (ECG) leads, a circumferential mapping catheter in the LSPV, and a decapolar catheter in the CS. In **Figure 2.3a**, activity in the CS is clearly disorganized with no consistent P-wave on the surface ECG. However, activity recorded within the vein is organized, suggesting limited connections from the LA. In **Figure 2.3b**, ablation targeting PV 4–5 results in a slowing of PV CL and a clear change in PV activation sequence. In **Figure 2.3c**, the recovered connection at PV 4–5 is targeted again to achieve sustained PV isolation. Note the low-amplitude far-field LAA activity recorded on the anterior aspect of the circumferential catheter in **Figure 2.3c**.

Left superior pulmonary vein isolation with atrial fibrillation confined inside the vein

Figure 2.4 shows termination of AF (star) and restoration of sinus rhythm by isolation of the LSPV. Arrhythmia continues within the vein. However, in the absence of a connection to the LA, sinus rhythm is maintained as evidenced by the surface ECG.

Note the dramatic change in activity recorded on the circumferential catheter from fractionated to regular PV tachycardia during AF compared with during sinus rhythm.

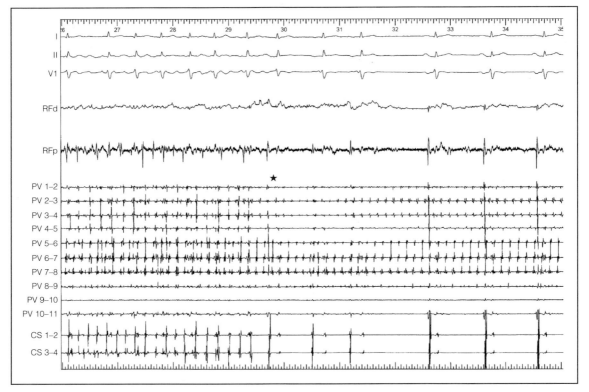

Figure 2.4. Left superior pulmonary vein isolation with atrial fibrillation confined inside the vein.
CS: coronary sinus; d: distal; PV: pulmonary vein; p: proximal; RF: ablation catheter.

Right superior pulmonary vein isolation with atrial fibrillation confined inside the vein

Figure 2.5a shows an ongoing irregular tachyarrhythmia within the PV, best seen in bipoles 7–8 and 8–9. The surface ECG has a P-wave morphology consistent with sinus rhythm. **Figure 2.5b** clearly demonstrates an association (arrows) between the prolonged local "gap" potential (star) recorded at LASSO bipole 1–2 and the surface P-wave. For the second and the fifth potentials recorded on PV bipole 1–2, conduction to the LA did not occur (interrupted lines), and no P-wave is seen on the surface ECG. This gap potential represents the site of breakthrough from the PV to the LA and explains the reason that targeting this site resulted in a subtle change in the surface P-wave (**Figure 2.5c**, star) and restoration of sinus rhythm.

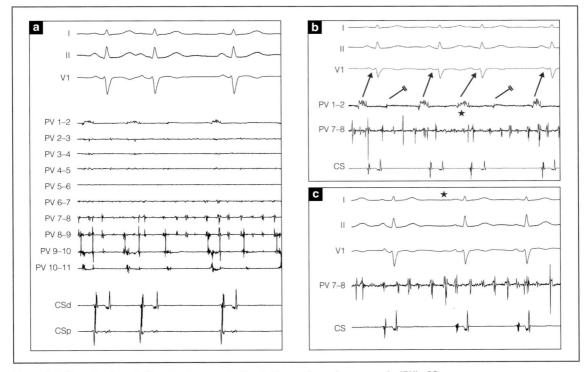

Figure 2.5. Pseudo sinus rhythm due to a gap in the right superior pulmonary vein (PV). CS: coronary sinus; d: distal; p: proximal.

3 | Electrogram-based ablation during disorganized left atrial activity

This chapter describes an approach to the electrically chaotic atrium and a systematic method whereby disorganized electrical activity can be rendered more organized, thereby facilitating electrogram interpretation.

- Chaotic activity

- Inferior left atrium/coronary sinus interface

- Inferior left atrium ablation

- Coronary sinus ablation

- Left atrial appendage ablation

- Septum

- Prolongation of atrial fibrillation cycle length during ablation of disorganized activity

Chaotic activity

After pulmonary vein (PV) isolation, atrial activity is often chaotic and too complex to allow analysis of the local cycle length (CL), morphology, or activation. Disorganized sites are ubiquitous in the left atrium (LA), and the first step in mapping is to determine the most favorable areas at which ablation will result in slowing and organization of global LA activity.

Continuous fractionated atrial electrograms (CFAEs) are defined as atrial electrograms (EGMs) with a CL of <120 ms that are composed of three deflections or more and/or have continuous electrical activity with no discernible isoelectric interval. Such activities may represent the ultimate degree of local electrical disorganization.

CFAEs can be described in terms of duration of continuous activity, degree of fractionation (representing the number of deflections of fractionated activity per unit time), absolute or mean voltage, and local mean CL.

In a recent study (Takahashi et al, 2008; *see* Bibliography), we found that continuous electrical activity is the local EGM morphology at which the impact of ablation is greatest, as determined by prolongation of the atrial fibrillation cycle length (AFCL) or termination of AF with predictive positive and negative values of 51% and 73%, respectively. Fractionation index, EGM voltage, and local mean CL are not significant predictors of effective sites for AF ablation.

Figure 3.1 depicts simultaneous EGM recordings from the ablation and coronary sinus (CS) catheters during AF. **Figure 3.1a** is a recording of continuous activity on the radiofrequency energy (RF) catheter without a return to baseline. **Figure 3.1b** shows a fractionated potential on the RF catheter with an interposed isoelectric interval. **Figure 3.1c** is an example of rapid activity recorded on the RF catheter with a frequency gradient to the CS. **Figure 3.1d** is an example of slow, low-voltage, fractionated activity.

Different underlying mechanisms may explain CFAEs. First, they may represent zones of colliding wave fronts or pivot points between different wavelets participating in the AF process. Second, their occurrence has been shown to be associated with prior acceleration of the AFCL. Finally, most fractionation is located at the periphery of sites of rapid activity, with a frequency gradient to surrounding atrial tissue.

However, given the ubiquitous presence of CFAE in persistent AF patients, the main issue is to distinguish active from passive patterns. It is critical to focus all possible effort on deciphering these chaotic intracardiac EGMs, as difficulty in their interpretation remains one of the major obstacles to efficacious ablation of persistent AF. From a purely anatomic perspective, ablation at the base of the left atrial appendage (LAA) and the interface between the inferior LA and CS has been shown to have the greatest impact on the AF process.

Figure 3.2 shows the completely chaotic activity in the posterior LA (A1–2 to E19–20) and the CS (CS 1–2 to CS 9–10). The posterior LA has been mapped with a five-spine catheter (PENTARAY). However, there is no discernible organization of activity to guide further mapping here. The inset NavX (St Jude Medical, Inc., MN, USA) electroanatomic fractionation map of the LA is shown in the posteroanterior view. The area of greatest fractionation (defined as a local CL of <120 ms) is the posterior LA, represented in white (*see* color scale). The least fractionated areas are represented as blue, while unfractionated areas are either purple or grey (representing scarring).

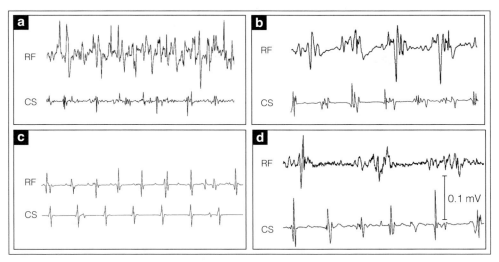

Figure 3.1. Chaotic activity. CS: coronary sinus; RF: ablation catheter.

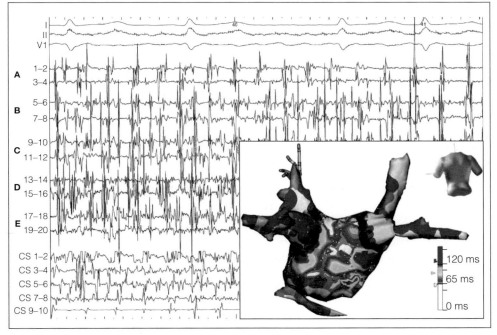

Figure 3.2. Chaotic activity in the posterior left atrium and coronary sinus (CS). The inset shows a NavX electroanatomic fractionation map of the left atrium (posteroanterior view).

Inferior left atrium/coronary sinus interface

The CS is a complex structure surrounded by a double muscular cuff formed during cardiac embryologic development. The first cuff is derived from the left horn of the sinus venosus and is in continuity with the right atrial musculature. The developing LA just adjacent to the CS gives rise to the second muscular cuff. These two muscular cuffs retain their interconnections during embryologic development. The portion that can be accessed endocardially is called the "inferior LA", while "CS" refers to the epicardial part.

Inferior LA ablation can generally be performed by looping the ablation catheter to increase stability. The tip is then dragged along the CS from septal to lateral positions (the segment between the 7 o'clock and the 4 o'clock positions in the left anterior oblique [LAO] projection) by withdrawing the catheter into the sheath (**Figures 3.3a–c**).

Ablation within the CS is started distally (approximately in the 4 o'clock position in the LAO projection) and pursued along the CS up to the ostium with the catheter tip deflected towards the LA (**Figures 3.3d–f**). This may help to minimize the risk of circumflex coronary artery injury. At the CS ostium, the catheter tip is deflected inferiorly to avoid injury to the atrioventricular (AV) node or fast pathway.

Figure 3.3 shows an anteroposterior fluoroscopic visualization of the catheter positions during ablation of the inferior LA (**Figures 3.3a–c**, endocardial) and CS (**Figures 3.3d–f**, epicardial). After looping the catheter into the LA facing the CS ostium (left) (**Figure 3.3a**), the catheter is then gradually withdrawn parallel to the CS along the posterior mitral annulus (MA) towards the lateral LA (**Figures 3.3b** and **c**). **Figures 3.3d–f** show the corresponding epicardial catheter positions at the ostial, middle, and distal segments, respectively, within the CS.

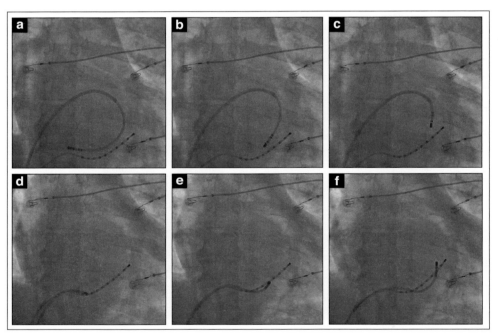

Figure 3.3. Anteroposterior fluoroscopic visualization of the catheter positions during ablation of the inferior left atrium and coronary sinus.

Inferior left atrium ablation

The dual composition of the CS musculature is reflected by the ablation results. The endpoint of ablation at the inferior LA is the elimination of local endocardial potentials and organization of chaotic activity recorded within the CS. Interruption of the muscular fascicles connecting the LA and the CS may explain the organization seen in CS activities, while longitudinal activation within the CS represents reduction of the inputs to this vessel from the LA (*see* inset line drawings in **Figure 3.4**).

Figure 3.4 shows the impact of endocardial ablation along the inferior LA on CS activation. Before ablation (**Figure 3.4a**), CS activation is inconsistent, chaotic, and continuous. With inferior LA ablation facing the proximal portion of the CS (**Figure 3.4b**, *see* artifact indicated by a star on CS 7–8), CS activation appears less chaotic and more consistent. Ablation facing the mid vessel (**Figure 3.4c**, *see* artifact indicated by a star on CS 5–6) further interrupts the connections between the LA and the CS such that, following ablation of the entire inferior LA (**Figure 3.4d**), there is organized activation. The CS drawings beneath **Figures 3.4a–d** illustrate the proposed mechanism to explain this phenomenon.

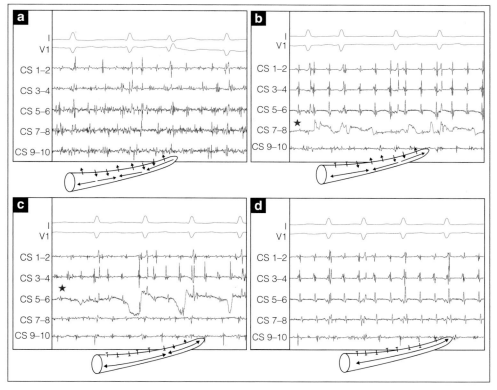

Figure 3.4. Inferior left atrium ablation. CS: coronary sinus.

Coronary sinus ablation

When complex and rapid EGMs remain within the CS after inferior LA ablation, RF energy is applied within the CS. This epicardial ablation directly targets the intrinsic CS musculature itself. The endpoint of ablation within the CS is local organization and slowing of electrical activities.

In our experience, ablation can be performed safely within the CS provided that the catheter tip is directed towards the LA and power is limited to 25 W with high irrigation rates (up to 60 mL/minute).

Complete disconnection of this structure is rarely necessary; it has not been demonstrated to provide additional clinical benefit in terms of outcome, and may carry a greater risk than ablation that aims only to achieve local organization and slowing. Therefore, a purposeful attempt to disconnect the CS should only be performed if focal ablation within the vessel fails to extinguish drivers originating from within.

Figure 3.5a shows the signals recorded from a decapolar catheter positioned within the CS following ablation of the endocardial aspect of the vessel (ie, the inferior LA). There is clear disorganization of activity with CFAEs in all leads, and continuous activity recorded on at least three of five bipoles. With ablation of the CS there is gradual organization of activity (**Figures 3.5b** and **c**). Note the contact artifacts in the distal and mid vessel (stars) as the ablation catheter is withdrawn from the distal-to-proximal CS. Following ablation at the endocardial and epicardial aspects of the CS, the complexity and amplitude of the locally recorded signals is greatly reduced (**Figure 3.5d**).

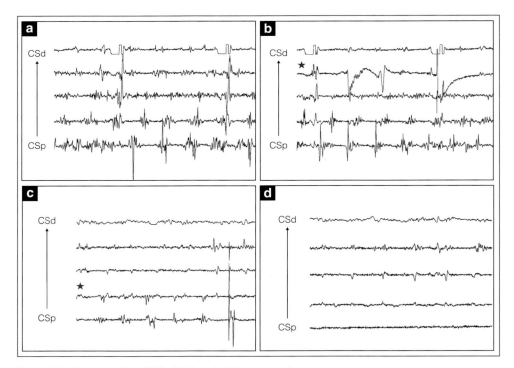

Figure 3.5. Coronary sinus (CS) ablation. d: distal; p: proximal.

Left atrial appendage ablation

All parts of the LAA may be implicated in perpetuation of AF. Ablation at this structure is guided by local EGM characteristics. In particular, the posterior ridge interposed between the left PVs and the mouth of the appendage often harbors complex activities and is routinely mapped.

Circumferential ablation of the LAA can be safely performed given the robust nature of its muscular connections. However, care must be taken to avoid electrical, and hence mechanical, disconnection of the LAA because of its role in LA function and the subsequent need for lifelong anticoagulation.

Figures 3.6a–c illustrate the effect of ablation at the posterior ridge of the LAA. The endpoint of ablation is organization of local activity by elimination of continuous fractionated EGMs (**Figure 3.6a**). Progressive organization of local activity at the base of the LAA can be appreciated from the RF catheter recordings (**Figures 3.6a–c**). The inset radiograph shows the transseptal sheath advanced to within the LAA, and the catheter inverted such that rotation of the sheath/catheter assembly can be used to target any disorganized activities mapped to the entire mouth of the LAA (*see* inset cartoon depiction of the LAA).

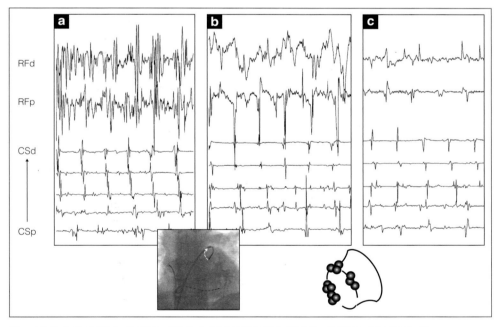

Figure 3.6. Left atrial appendage ablation: **(a)** fractionated; **(b)** intermediate; **(c)** organized. RF: ablation catheter; CS: coronary sinus; d: distal; p: proximal.

Septum

The interatrial septum is anatomically defined as the fossa ovalis and its rim. It is often an area of highly complex activity. To reach the septum, a small loop of the ablation catheter can be made to move back towards the fossa ovalis, as illustrated in **Figure 3.7**.

Figure 3.7a is an anteroposterior radiographic projection showing the ablation catheter looped within the LA such that the tip is brought close to the inferior aspect of the interatrial septum. With further flexion and withdrawal of the catheter (**Figure 3.7b**), more of the fossa can be reached. In this patient, continuous complex electrical activity was recorded by the ablation catheter positioned at a septal site (**Figure 3.7c**, Sept); ablation here restored sinus rhythm (**Figure 3.7d**).

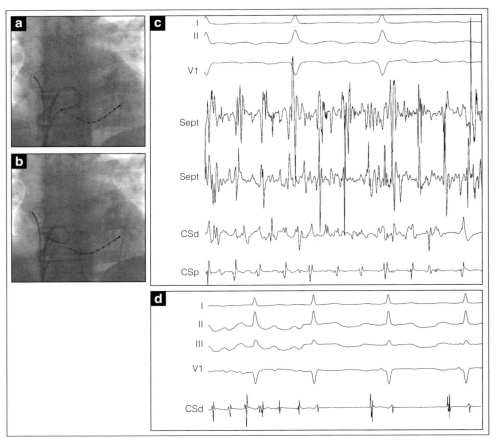

Figure 3.7. Septal ablation. CS: coronary sinus; d: distal; p: proximal; Sept: septum.

Prolongation of atrial fibrillation cycle length during ablation of disorganized activity

The initial AFCL has been shown to be the strongest predictor of success for AF ablation. An AFCL of <140 ms is associated with AF termination in <69% of cases, while a higher AFCL is associated with a >89% likelihood of AF termination.

As illustrated in **Figure 3.8**, the impact of ablation in each region during EGM-based ablation can be quantified in both atria by simultaneous AFCL monitoring. After each step of ablation, a gradual prolongation of AFCL is observed (a change in AFCL of >6 ms is considered significant).

Conversion to sinus rhythm or atrial tachycardia (AT) occurs when the AFCL reaches 180–200 ms and, conversely, rarely occurs when the AFCL is shorter. Prolongation of the AFCL is accompanied by organization of complex atrial activities, permitting discrete mapping.

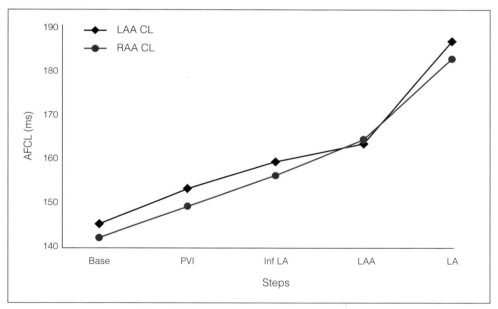

Figure 3.8. The impact of ablation of each region during electrogram-based ablation, as measured by atrial fibrillation cycle length (AFCL) monitoring. CL: cycle length; Inf LA: inferior left atrium; LA: left atrium; LAA: left atrial appendage; PVI: pulmonary vein isolation; RAA: right atrial appendage.

4 | Electrogram-based ablation during organized left atrial activity

This chapter describes how to recognize patterns of activation during atrial fibrillation once disorganized activity has been organized by catheter ablation.

- Mapping of organized atrial fibrillation

- Localized temporal gradient

- Centrifugal activity

- Rapid activity

- Sites of rapid activity and fractionation

- Pseudo rapid activity

- Localized re-entrant fibrillating source

Mapping of organized atrial fibrillation

Atrial fibrillation may be described as organized when there is clear evidence of atrial fibrillation (AF), ie, beat-to-beat cycle length (CL) variation of >20 ms, but also clear evidence of stability of activation sequence. We have defined the latter property as a consistent intra-atrial activation sequence for more than 75% of a 10-minute observation window, and in which there are predominantly discrete atrial electrograms rather than complex, fractionated electrograms.

Localized sources perpetuating AF have been evidenced during ablation procedures by persistent fibrillatory activity confined within isolated left atrial (LA) areas after restoration of sinus rhythm. These sources play an important role in AF maintenance, in addition to pulmonary vein (PV) activity and re-entrant loops. After pulmonary vein isolation (PVI) and linear lesions, ablation of these sources remains the last step of substrate elimination and results in atrial tachycardia (AT) conversion or restoration of sinus rhythm.

A localized source may be a discrete point or a small area. When mapping of atrial activation during organized AF converges towards an origin of activity, a small area displaying centrifugal activation and including the localized source can be analyzed.

This area may include a discrete point (harboring <75% of the CL), which allows tracking of the earliest activity. Local electrograms (EGMs) display centrifugal activation with or without 1:1 conduction to the adjacent atrium (same or faster CL of the source compared with AFCL, respectively).

In the majority of cases, the source is not a discrete point but a small area. This area of earliest activation displays electrical activity covering 75–100% of the CL, suggesting a localized small circuit. By mapping with a conventional quadripolar ablation catheter, local potentials will display either continuous activity spanning most of the CL, or temporally alternating potentials between distal and proximal bipoles (depending on the re-entrant circuit size and properties). By mapping with a high-density 20-pole catheter, local activity will span most or all of the CL.

Figure 4.1 illustrates the human heart laid open from behind, with the LA to the left and the RA to the right. Three separate arrhythmogenic mechanisms are illustrated here with wave-front propagation illustrated by the arrows:

- Localized re-entry at site **a**.

- Focal activation with 1:1 conduction from a dead-end structure (superior vena cava; SVC) at site **b** (star).

- A focal source with centrifugal activation of the surrounding atrial tissue at site **c** (star).

At site **a**, there is a hypothetical re-entrant circuit in the posterior LA. When the mapping catheter is placed over this area, the EGM shown in **Figure 4.1a$_1$** is recorded, illustrating a temporal gradient of activation between the proximal and distal bipoles. Positioning of a multipolar mapping catheter at this site (**Figure 4.1a$_2$**) shows that the entire CL of activity may be recorded at two catheter spines (A1–4 and B5–8, highlighted in pink shading), with consistent activation of the remaining catheter spines thereby providing strong support for a localized re-entrant circuit.

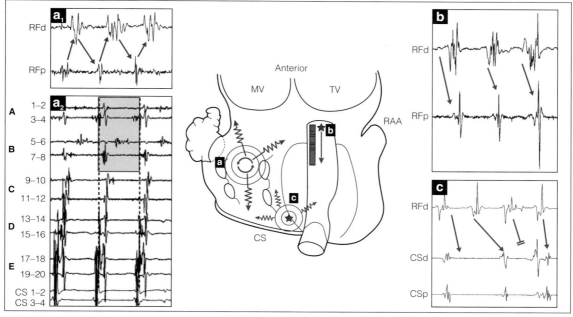

Figure 4.1. A line drawing of the human heart laid open from behind. **(a–c)** Mapping at sites a–c. CS: coronary sinus; d: distal; MV: mitral valve; p: proximal; RAA: right atrial appendage; RF: ablation catheter; TV: tricuspid valve. The stars indicate the origin of focal activity.

When the mapping catheter is aligned with the distal bipole nearest a focal source within the SVC, there is consistent activation from distal to proximal position (**Figure 4.1b**), provided 1:1 conduction from source to atrium is maintained.

Figure 4.1c illustrates rapid activity recorded at the mapping catheter positioned within the LA, but without 1:1 conduction to the coronary sinus (CS) – ie, a frequency gradient exists between these two sites that can be exploited to map the origin of centrifugal activation.

Localized temporal gradient

Ablation at the site of an activation gradient of >70 ms between the proximal and distal electrode bipoles is associated with AF slowing or termination. This pattern may represent the sequential atrial activation occurring at the periphery of rotating waves, ie, localized re-entry, and this may maintain either AF or AT depending on the rotor velocity and the electrical properties of the atrium.

Although a temporal gradient can also occur by chance in the case of slow conduction, a consistent gradient, together with centrifugal activation to the surrounding atrium, suggests that the catheter is crossing a localized re-entrant circuit.

The case in **Figure 4.2** illustrates the importance of recognizing a temporal gradient pattern with the quadripolar ablation catheter during mapping of organized AF. The ablation catheter is straddling a localized re-entrant circuit with a temporal gradient of activation recorded between both bipoles (arrows). Note that there is no clearly discernible P-wave on the surface electrocardiogram (ECG), and that there is a subtle change in the delay between

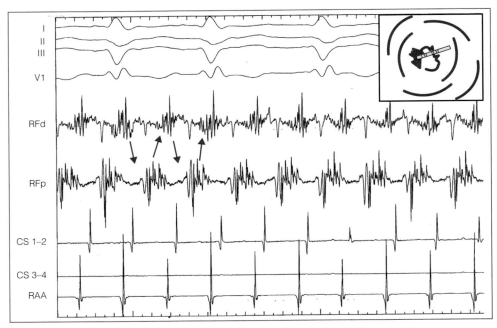

Figure 4.2. Localized temporal gradient. The inset cartoon depicts the ablation catheter spanning the local re-entrant circuit. CS: coronary sinus; d: distal; p: proximal; RAA: right atrial appendage; RF: ablation catheter.

the right atrial appendage (RAA) and the CS, consistent with AF rather than AT. Ablation at this site resulted in termination of AF by conversion to a stable CL AT within 20 seconds of ablation.

Centrifugal activity

Initially, mapping of organized AF requires determination of the LA area from which the centrifugal activation emanates. This is followed by high-density mapping within that area to determine the precise site of earliest activity, and whether that site represents a focal point or a localized re-entry.

EGMs localized in the area of earliest activity may display centrifugal activation with 1:1 conduction to the adjacent atrium (same CL as the source compared with AFCL).

The case in **Figure 4.3** illustrates organized AF with a consistent sequence inside the CS, with centrifugal activity coming from its mid part (arrows) and spreading out to the surrounding tissue. On the basis of this one trace, it is not possible to say whether the CS or the inferior LA is the culprit site. However, ablation at the site of earliest activity (mid CS) converted AF to AT, implicating the CS in the fibrillatory process.

Multipolar contact mapping catheters may be used for the characterization of sites of centrifugal activation. The catheter schema (**Figure 4.4**, inset) shows a centrifugal source (star) activating all spines of the catheter from the proximal to distal position. The real-time EGMs are seen in the main illustration. There is proximal-to-distal activation on spines A–E, as indicated by the direction of the arrows. This site may represent a focal source of endocardial activation.

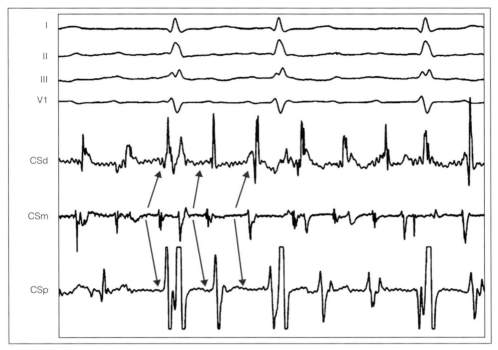

Figure 4.3. Centrifugal activity in a case showing organized atrial fibrillation with a consistent sequence inside the coronary sinus (CS); d: distal; m: mid; p: proximal.

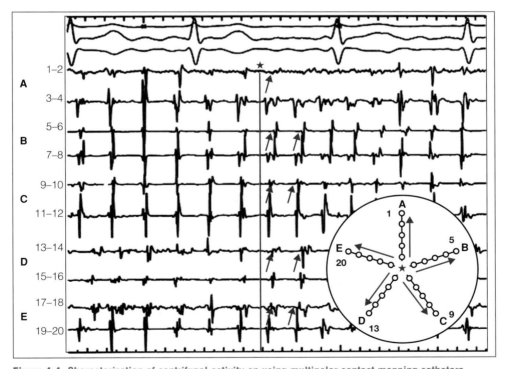

Figure 4.4. Characterization of centrifugal activity on using multipolar contact mapping catheters.

Rapid activity

Figure 4.5 depicts a source of rapid activity within the CS (local CL of 114 ms), with distal-to-proximal activation and without 1:1 conduction to the recording site in the left atrial appendage (LAA; local CL of 220 ms).

Ablation within the distal CS terminated AF and restored sinus rhythm. Note the sinus rhythm P-wave giving rise to a consistent activation in the CS (arrows), but with ongoing dissociated CS activity (stars).

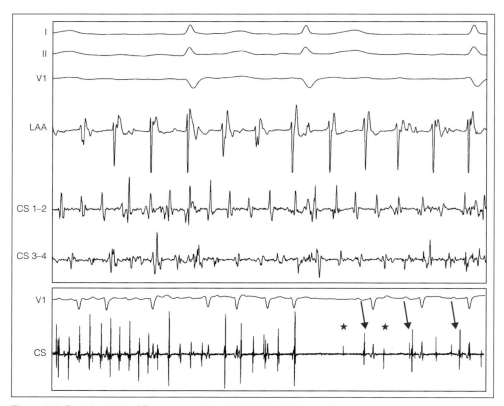

Figure 4.5. Rapid activity. CS: coronary sinus; LAA: left atrial appendage.

Sites of rapid activity and fractionation

This case illustrates an approach to the evaluation of fractionation recorded at the posterior wall of the LA. Once fractionation was recognized (**Figure 4.6a**), mapping of the tissue surrounding the area of fractionation showed more rapid local activity, with a distal-to-proximal activation pattern on the ablation catheter (**Figure 4.6b**).

In the absence of a fixed timing reference (non-1:1 conduction to the CS), the catheter is moved over the suspected site of rapid activity. When a distal-to-proximal activation sequence converts to a proximal-to-distal sequence, the catheter has passed the epicenter of activation, and indicates the optimal site for ablation.

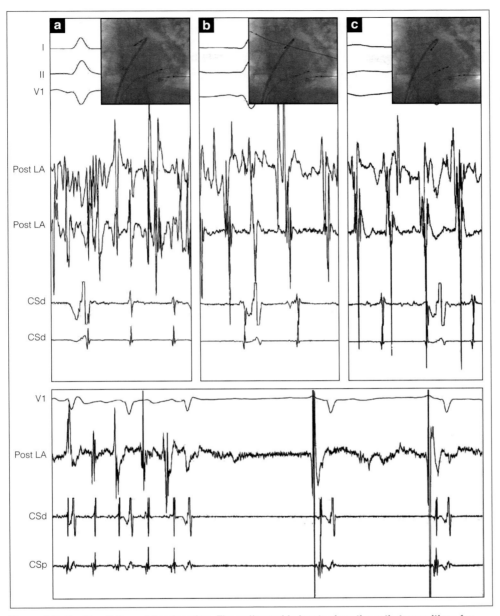

Figure 4.6. Rapid activity and fractionation. The radiographic insets show the catheter positions for each of the ablation signals recorded in panels **a–c**. CS: coronary sinus; d: distal; LA: left atrium; p: proximal; Post: posterior.

Ablation targeting the site of earliest and most rapid activity (**Figure 4.6c**) was successful in terminating AF (lowest panel), ie, the last site before a change in the activation sequence on the ablation catheter. In this case, fractionation is likely to represent a passive phenomenon, best explained by slow conduction at the outer limit of the region displaying the most rapid, regular activity.

Pseudo rapid activity

In mapping sources of rapid activity, it is important to distinguish between true rapid activity and slower activity with double potentials secondary to functional conduction block.

Figure 4.7a shows a spontaneous change in the locally recorded potential, from a single discrete potential to a double potential (star) at the same site. **Figure 4.7b** is a later recording from the same site. The double potentials are equally split, giving the false impression of locally rapid activity.

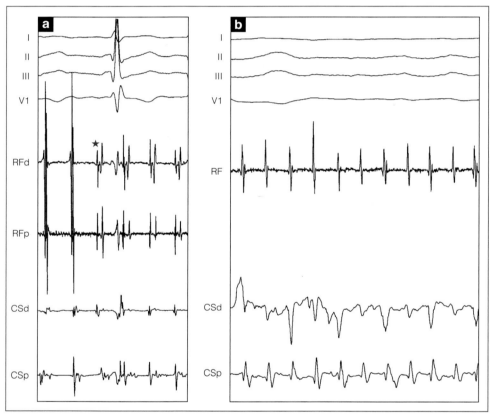

Figure 4.7. Pseudo rapid activity. CS: coronary sinus; d: distal; p: proximal; RF: ablation catheter.

Localized re-entrant fibrillating source

In the case of a localized source displaying re-entrant properties, sequential mapping with the distal bipole of the ablation catheter within the area of interest can also be performed to track different parts of the CL, as illustrated in **Figure 4.8**.

Prior mapping showed that endocardial LA activation was organized with a consistent septal-to-lateral and high-to-low activation sequence in the anterior LA, and a low-to-high sequence in the posterior LA (red arrows).

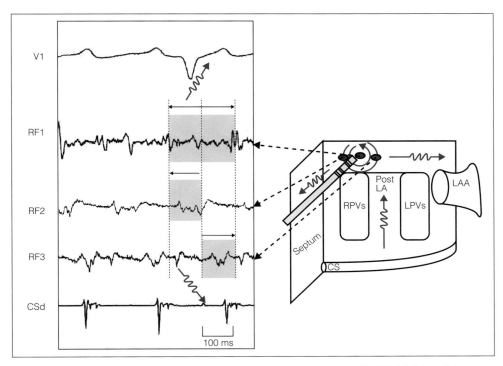

Figure 4.8. Localized re-entrant fibrillating source. CS: coronary sinus; d: distal; LAA: left atrial appendage; LPV: left pulmonary vein; Post LA: posterior left atrium; RF: ablation catheter; RPV: right pulmonary vein.

The ablation catheter was placed anterior and septal to the roof line. At this position, within a small area, EGMs recorded activity spanning the entire cardiac cycle (pink shading, radiofrequency energy [RF] 1), the initial part of the CL (pink shading, RF2), and the later part of the CL (pink shading, RF3). These recordings were made sequentially, but are displayed under each other here to facilitate understanding.

These findings were most compatible with a localized re-entrant circuit (bold circular arrow) from which the remainder of the LA is activated centrifugally. Note that the posterior wall is activated from inferior to superior because of conduction block at the roof line. Ablation at the site of this circuit slowed and then terminated the tachycardia. The completeness of block at the roof line was confirmed in sinus rhythm.

5 | Right atrial ablation

This chapter describes an approach to ablation of the right atrium in the event that left atrial ablation fails to terminate atrial fibrillation.

- Right atrial ablation

- Right atrial appendage ablation

- Intercaval region

- Entire circuit within localized area in lateral right atrium

- Superior vena cava

Right atrial ablation

In 15% of patients with persistent atrial fibrillation (AF), sinus rhythm cannot be restored by ablation in the left atrium (LA). In these patients, the presence of perpetuators in the right atrium (RA) should be considered.

This situation is expected when, during LA ablation, only a relative prolongation of the cycle length (CL) occurs in the RA: a shorter AFCL by 15–20 ms in the right atrial appendage (RAA) compared with in the left atrial appendage (LAA) would suggest that the RA might harbor the perpetuating influence for ongoing AF. Similarly, pauses in activity in the LA electrograms (EGMs), without corresponding pauses in the RA EGMs, would suggest the RA as the culprit chamber.

The approach to mapping (ie, organization of chaotic activity and mapping of organized AF) and the EGM targets within the RA are the same as for the LA. Preferential anatomic areas at which there is a higher incidence of AF termination during ablation are the RAA, the intercaval region, the superior vena cava (SVC), and the coronary sinus (CS) ostium.

Figures 5.1a and **b** illustrate the change in AFCL recorded in both appendages during ablation in two separate patients. In **Figure 5.1a**, there is a parallel increase in the AFCL in both chambers with increasing LA ablation. In **Figure 5.1b**, there is a right-to-left frequency gradient at the outset, and a much steeper increase in LAA CL than that recorded in the RAA with increasing ablation. This is consistent with an important role for the RA in driving AF in this patient. **Figure 5.1c** demonstrates a frequency gradient from the RAA to the CS. There is ongoing activity in the RAA during a pause in CS activity (star), implying that, at this moment, there is likely to be a driving influence within the RA.

Right atrial appendage ablation

The circumferential mapping catheter can be used to map the RAA and guide ablation towards the sites of most rapid or earliest activity. Ablation at the superior part of this structure results in conversion to atrial tachycardia (AT), implying the presence of a local driving influence during AF.

In **Figure 5.2**, the inset radiographic image shows the circumferential mapping catheter in the RAA and the ablation catheter at the upper margin of the RAA. In **Figure 5.2a**, there is already a degree of organization of AF, but with rapid and fractionated activity seen in poles 4–7, which corresponds to the septal and superior aspects of the RAA. Ablation at these poles organized, slowed, and then terminated AF. Note the variable RAA to CS conduction in **Figure 5.2a**. This organizes in **Figure 5.2b** to a 1:1 relationship.

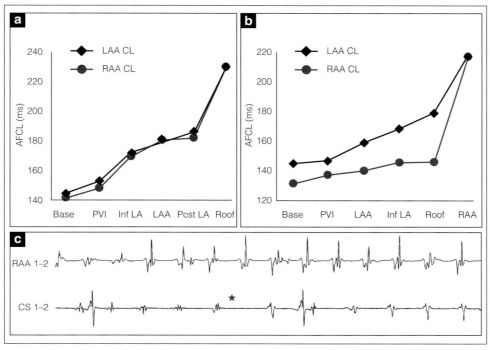

Figure 5.1. Atrial fibrillation cycle length (AFCL) changes during right atrial ablation. CL: cycle length; Inf LA: inferior left atrium; LAA: left atrial appendage; Post LA: posterior left atrium; PVI: pulmonary vein isolation; RAA: right atrial appendage.

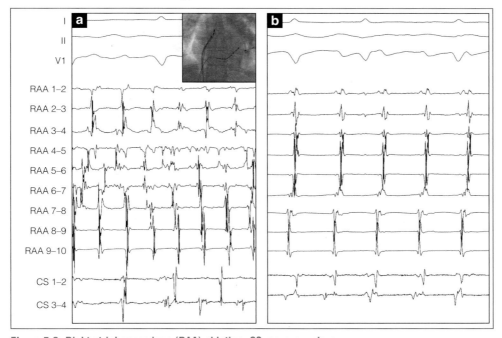

Figure 5.2. Right atrial appendage (RAA) ablation. CS: coronary sinus.

Intercaval region

The intercaval aspect of the RA represents a site of fibrillatory activity that is easily targeted for ablation. Using the EGM-guided parameters described earlier, ablation can be performed by dragging the catheter facing posteriorly from the SVC to the inferior vena cava (IVC), again with local organization and slowing as the ablation endpoints. It is not intended to form a complete posterior line of conduction block between the SVC and the IVC.

In the example shown in **Figure 5.3**, conversion from AF to AT occurred during intercaval ablation. The variable CL activity on the left of **Figure 5.3** is replaced by regular activity with a consistent proximal-to-distal activation sequence in the CS.

It is interesting to note also that there is a pause in the activity recorded in the CS without a corresponding pause at the posterior RA (intercaval ablation site – radiofrequency energy distal [RFd]) or the RAA, suggesting the presence of a driver within the RA.

Although there are no distinguishing features recorded on the radiofrequency energy (RF) catheter, incessant changes in the activation pattern do not permit source mapping. Occasionally, when all else fails, it is necessary to be guided to anatomic sites that have not been previously ablated.

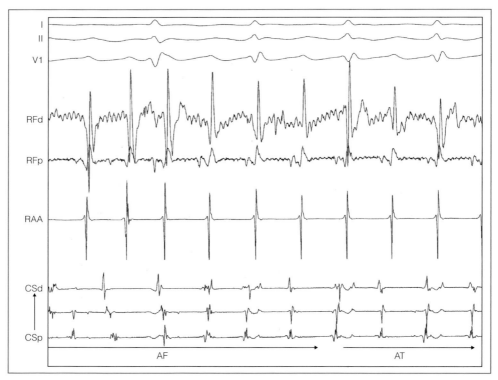

Figure 5.3. Conversion from atrial fibrillation (AF) to atrial tachycardia (AT) during intercaval ablation. CS: coronary sinus; d: distal; p: proximal; RAA: right atrial appendage; RF: ablation catheter.

Entire circuit within localized area in lateral right atrium

As described for the LA, small circuits may be mapped within the RA. The ablation of these circuits impacts on the fibrillatory process.

During the phase of mapping of organized AF, once the AFCL has been sufficiently prolonged, centrifugal activity may be demonstrated at the center of which discrete sites can be identified where activity spanning >70% of the fibrillatory CL is seen. Mapping of adjacent areas will often reveal activities spanning adjoining parts of the CL, consistent with local re-entrant activation.

In the example shown in **Figure 5.4a**, the RAA and CS EGMs were recorded simultaneously, while the RA 1–3 EGMs were recorded sequentially. They have been displayed one under the other to emphasize the technique of localized mapping to define a localized re-entrant circuit with centrifugal activation of the atrium (curved arrows; **Figure 5.4b)**. The RA 1 EGM was recorded from the most superior site, as indicated on the schematic of the RA (**Figure 5.4b**), and recorded activity from the second half of the cycle (pink-shaded area). The RA 2 EGM shows continuous fractionation and was recorded close to the centre point.

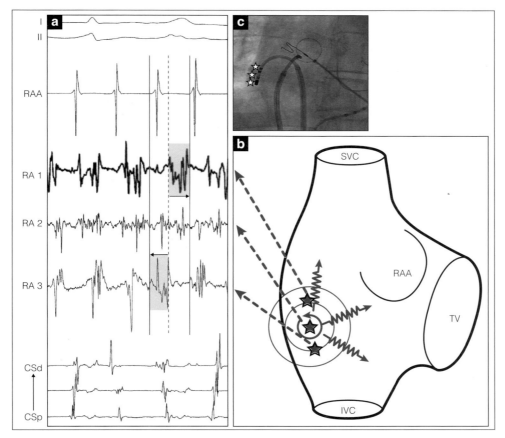

Figure 5.4. Entire circuit within localized area in lateral right atrium. CS: coronary sinus; d: distal; IVC: inferior vena cava; p: proximal; RA: right atrium; RAA: right atrial appendage; SVC: superior vena cava; TV: tricuspid valve.

The RA 3 EGM was recorded from the most inferior position and shows activity from the first half of the cycle (pink-shaded area). Here, the entire CL of activation can be mapped to a small region in the low lateral RA, as illustrated by the arrows within the pink-shaded areas. Ablation at this site terminated AF. The inset shows an anteroposterior radiographic projection with a circumferential catheter in the RAA and the ablation catheter position in the lateral RA **(Figure 5.4c)**. The stars represent the sites of recording.

Superior vena cava

The SVC has been implicated as an ectopic source in the initiation of paroxysmal AF. Its role in persistent AF is less well defined. However, in our experience, it is rarely the site of AF termination by ablation and should only be targeted for isolation if a focal source can be demonstrated within. Therefore, in our laboratory, it is not a routine part of the approach to catheter ablation of persistent AF.

The X-ray image in **Figure 5.5** shows the mapping catheter at the SVC–RA junction. The decapolar catheter is inverted such that the distal poles lie inferiorly and the proximal poles superiorly. **Figure 5.5a** demonstrates a distal-to-proximal activation sequence at the ablation catheter (indicated by the red and the white arrows), consistent with activation exiting rather than entering the SVC. The RA is activated in a craniocaudal direction (decapolar catheter activates from proximal to distal, as shown by the red and the white arrows). Ablation at the SVC–RA junction terminated AF by conversion to AT **(Figure 5.5b)**.

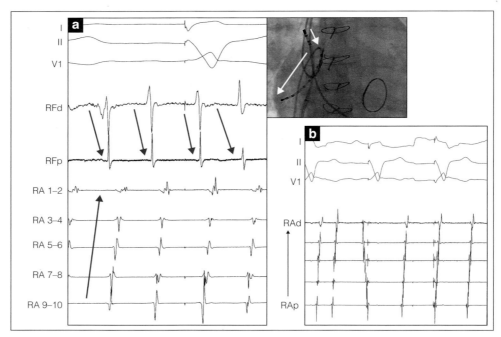

Figure 5.5. Ablation at the superior vena cava. d: distal; p: proximal; RA: right atrium; RF: ablation catheter.

6 | Ablation of other structures

In this chapter, structures less commonly involved in the initiation and maintenance of atrial fibrillation will be described, including the vein of Marshall and the left-sided superior vena cava. These are included as interesting illustrations of how basic electrophysiological principles can be used to evaluate activities recorded at any point within the heart.

- Vein of Marshall

- Left superior vena cava

Vein of Marshall

Figure 6.1a is a radiograph of the coronary sinus (CS) taken during a contrast injection. The vein of Marshall (VOM) is readily visualized, originating from the posterior left atrium (LA) close to the ostium of the left inferior pulmonary vein (LIPV) and the base of the left atrial appendage (LAA). There is a five-spine catheter (PENTARAY) close to the ostium of the left inferior pulmonary vein (LIPV). Here, the star over the CS catheter corresponds to the electrogram (EGM) recording on the CS catheter. The second star over the distal poles of the PENTARAY catheter corresponds to the distal pole recording (PRd), and the star over the proximal bipole of the PENTARAY corresponds to the proximal pole recording (PRp).

In this orientation, the spine facing inferiorly has recorded a larger ventricular EGM peak in the distal (PRd) than in the proximal (PRp) position. Bipole 3–4 of the decapole (distal coronary sinus; CSd) has recorded the largest ventricular EGM peak, as it is closest to the left ventricle, but immediately after the ventricular electrogram is a small, sharp potential (star) that is recorded on the distal and then the proximal bipole of the arm of interest on the PENTARAY catheter (**Figure 6.1b**). We hypothesized that this represented a slowly conducting VOM (curved arrow). This was proven by recording a continuous potential from proximal to distal within the VOM using a 5 Fr bipole, bridging the earliest and latest potentials recorded (**Figures 6.1c** and **d**, wavy arrow).

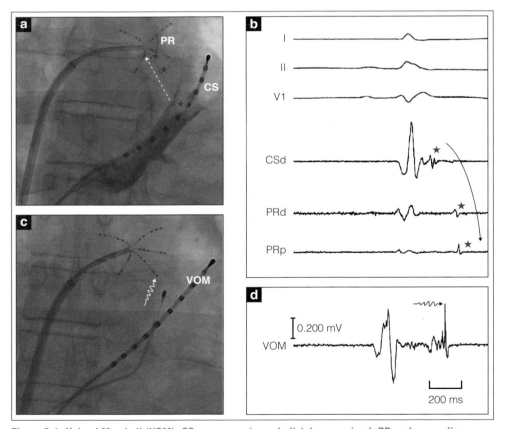

Figure 6.1. Vein of Marshall (VOM). CS: coronary sinus; d: distal; p: proximal; PR: pole recording.

Ablation at the ostium of the vein abolished the bridging potential and resulted in the disappearance of all late potentials. This suggests that the VOM was being activated very late and slowly, and via the CS.

Left superior vena cava

A persistent left superior vena cava (LSVC) has been well described as a trigger for atrial fibrillation and a source of atrial tachycardia (AT). It is a formidable target for ablation as it is usually very large and runs parallel to the LA, perhaps with a greater potential for communication with the LA than is the case for the normal CS.

The radiograph in **Figure 6.2a** is a venogram of the persistent LSVC using an NIH catheter (Cordis Corporation, Miami, FL, USA). The radiograph in **Figure 6.2b** illustrates how a circumferential mapping catheter may be used to guide isolation of this vessel at the ostium.

The elimination of the connections to the LA is critically important. This can be performed as previously described, ie, by endocardial ablation along the inferior LA and further ablation within the LSVC, with the catheter directed towards the LA.

The EGMs (**Figure 6.2c**) show the site of earliest activity on the circumferential mapping catheter closer to the CS ostium (star). Activation spreads from proximal to distal positions and the quadripolar catheter records the latest local activity, shortly after the left atrial EGM.

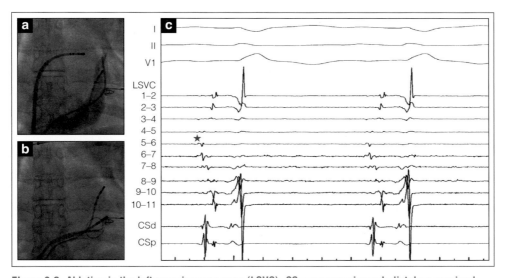

Figure 6.2. Ablation in the left superior vena cava (LSVC). CS: coronary sinus; d: distal; p: proximal.

7 | Linear lesions

This chapter describes the techniques for ablation and assessment of conduction block across linear lesions at the left atrial roof and the mitral and tricuspid isthmuses.

- Linear ablation

- Roof line

- Roof-line ablation during atrial fibrillation

- Assessment of roof-line block

- Mitral isthmus line

- Mitral isthmus line ablation during atrial fibrillation

- Mitral isthmus line ablation during sinus rhythm

- Assessment of mitral isthmus line block

- Assessment of combined mitral isthmus block and roof-line block

- Cavotricuspid isthmus ablation during atrial fibrillation

- Cavotricuspid isthmus block assessment

Linear ablation

Linear ablation is an important tool in the ablation of atrial fibrillation (AF). Not only does it target large areas of atrial tissue, but it is also critical for treatment of the atrial tachycardias (ATs) seen during both index and follow-up procedures.

The efficacy of linear ablation lesions may be related in part to an interruption of wavelets and macro re-entries, but also to an alteration of autonomic innervation, atrial debulking, and the organization or abolition of local complex electrograms (EGMs).

The left atrial roof and lateral mitral isthmus are the most common sites for linear ablation in this context.

Roof line

Because linear ablation at the left atrial roof is performed by connecting the margins of both superior pulmonary veins (PVs), its length depends on the extent of the PV encircling lesions. Complete block can be achieved in 96% of cases with an average of 12 ± 6 minutes of radiofrequency energy (RF) delivery.

The line is preferentially performed at the most cranial part of the left atrium (LA) to minimize the risk of esophageal injury. Three different approaches can be applied:

- Perpendicular to the roof (with a reduced power of 25 W to minimize the likelihood of steam pop and perforation).

- Parallel to the roof, with the sheath pointing towards the left atrial appendage (LAA) and the catheter towards the right superior pulmonary vein (RSPV), or *vice versa*.

- Occasionally, by looping the catheter 360° in the LA so that the tip is pointing towards the left superior pulmonary vein (LSPV).

In the less aggressive parallel orientations, up to 30 W can be used. Higher irrigation rates may be required due to occlusion of the irrigation holes by this orientation.

Figure 7.1 shows catheter orientations used for ablation of the roof line. The left three panels (**Figure 7.1a**) demonstrate three techniques for ablating the right margin of the line (the top panel shows the catheter perpendicular to the roof, the middle panel has the catheter parallel to the roof, and the bottom panel shows looping of the catheter). The panels of **Figure 7.1b** demonstrate how to ablate the middle of the roof, and the panels of **Figure 7.1c** demonstrate how to target the left margin of the line. The arrows in the middle panels indicate the direction of motion of the sheath and therefore the catheter tip. In the bottom panel of **Figure 7.1c**, retraction of the catheter into the sheath will result in movement of the catheter tip from the LSPV towards the RSPV, ie, in the direction of the white arrow.

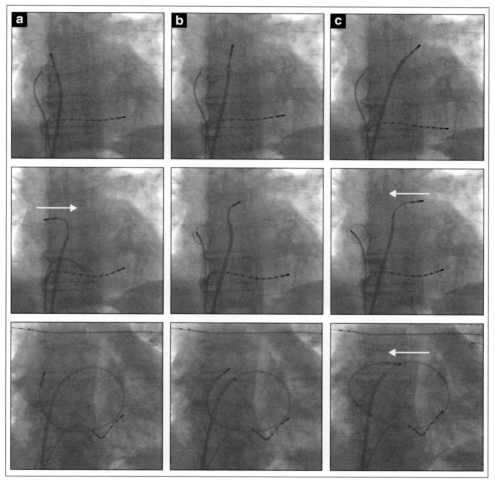

Figure 7.1. Ablation of the roof line.

Roof-line ablation during atrial fibrillation

During roof-line ablation in AF, the endpoint is the elimination of local EGMs. **Figure 7.2** illustrates three steps of roof-line ablation during AF, with first complex continuous EGMs followed by slowing and organizing of EGMs and then elimination.

The panels show the EGMs recorded at the LA roof, within the CS (distal and proximal), and within the right atrial appendage (RAA). In **Figure 7.2a**, prior to ablation at the roof, there is highly fractionated, continuous activity, with more organized activity recorded in the CS and RAA. With ablation at the LA roof, there is an initial organization of activity, with elimination of the continuous component of the complex activity recorded prior to ablation (**Figure 7.2b**). With further ablation (**Figure 7.2c**), there is complete elimination of activity along the trajectory of the roof line and prolongation of the cycle length (CL) recorded at two remote sites.

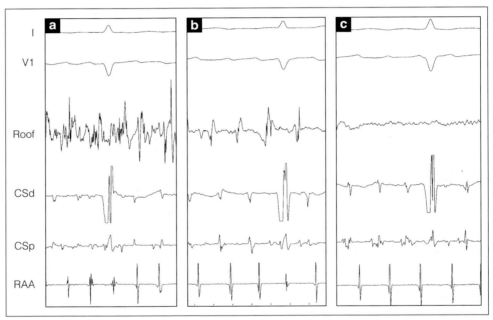

Figure 7.2. Roof-line ablation during atrial fibrillation. CS: coronary sinus; d: distal; p: proximal; RAA: right atrial appendage.

Assessment of roof-line block

Following ablation, a complete line of conduction block is confirmed in sinus rhythm. **Figure 7.3a** illustrates the principles behind assessment of the roof line. In this example, a deflectable quadripolar catheter has been advanced to the LAA, from where pacing can be performed. A decapolar catheter was positioned perpendicular to the roof line.

Without conduction block at the roof line, pacing of the LAA should result in parallel wave fronts of activation from the inferior and superior LA (white arrows), as the left PVs are circumnavigated, colliding on the posterior wall.

When the roof line is blocked, there should be no wave front from above, and therefore, all activation of the posterior LA should proceed from inferior to superior (from position 1 to positions 2 and 3). Furthermore, the posterior LA is activated from left (2) to right (3) if the mitral isthmus is not blocked.

Figure 7.3b shows the EGMs recorded with the decapolar catheter in the orientation shown in **Figure 7.3a**, ie, straddling the line with the proximal poles anterior and the distal poles posterior to the line. During LAA pacing, potentials can be recorded from both sides of the line as the decapolar catheter crosses it (illustrated by arrows in panel **b**).

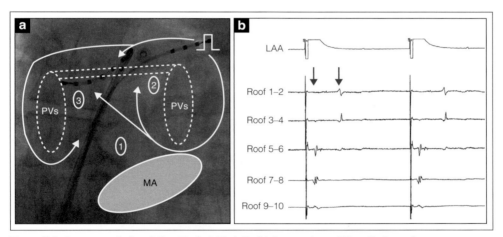

Figure 7.3. Assessment of roof-line block. LAA: left atrial appendage; MA: mitral annulus; PV: pulmonary vein.

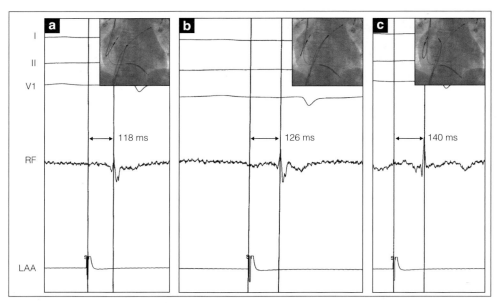

Figure 7.4. Assessment of roof-line block. LAA: left atrial appendage; RF: ablation catheter.

The tracings in **Figure 7.4** illustrate assessment of roof-line block. Usually, we position the CS catheter in the LAA for pacing and use the RF catheter to evaluate activation of the posterior LA. The posterior LA is activated from low (**Figure 7.4a**) to high (**Figures 7.4b** and **c**) and from left (**Figure 7.4b**) to right (**Figure 7.4c**) when the mitral isthmus line is not blocked. The inset radiographic images (**a–c**) indicate at annotated intervals the delay recorded from stimulus artifact to local EGM at the recording position (ablation catheter).

If the CS catheter cannot be advanced through the transseptal puncture, evaluation of the posterior LA activation can be reliably performed during sinus rhythm, during anterior RA pacing (as close as possible to the septum), or during pacing of the pulmonary artery. However, there is less accuracy given the distance to the line of block. In these cases, an ascending wave front in the posterior wall can also be demonstrated.

Mitral isthmus line

Ablation of the mitral isthmus line is the most challenging step in the process of persistent AF ablation and is therefore the last step of LA ablation. Block can be achieved in only approximately 90% of cases, and failure can have proarrhythmic consequences. Furthermore, there is a 1–2% risk of periprocedural tamponade.

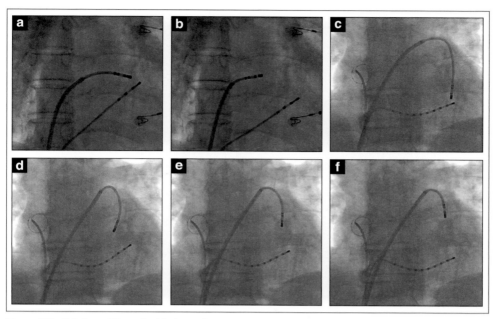

Figure 7.5. Ablation of the mitral isthmus line.

Ablation of the mitral isthmus starts at the lateral mitral isthmus. The sheath and catheter are rotated clockwise to extend the lesion posteriorly to the ostium of the left inferior pulmonary vein (LIPV). During this movement, the ablation catheter is progressively pulled back into the sheath (**Figures 7.5a** and **b**). Another approach parallel to the line is possible, allowing higher power. However, this requires the sheath to be advanced to the LAA ostium to obtain stability (**Figures 7.5c** and **d**).

It is often necessary to extend the line to the base of the LAA (**Figures 7.5e** and **f**) and inside the CS (with power limited to 25 W) in up to 80% of cases in order to achieve isthmus block.

Mitral isthmus line ablation during atrial fibrillation

Linear ablation is performed on a purely anatomic basis during AF, as the variability of CL means that it is not possible to follow the development of double potentials and conduction delay as the ablation proceeds. The same is true for the roof line and the cavotricuspid isthmus (CTI) line. Nevertheless, the endpoint of ablation during AF remains the same and is electrophysiologically guided: elimination of local EGMs along the trajectory of the line connecting two electrically inactive sites, ie, the mitral valve annulus and the encircling lesion around the LIPV.

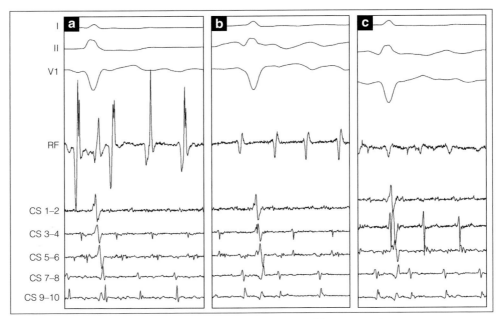

Figure 7.6. Mitral isthmus line ablation during atrial fibrillation. CS: coronary sinus; RF: ablation catheter.

It is rare to achieve conduction block across the mitral isthmus without further ablation once AF has been terminated by conversion to AT or to sinus rhythm. **Figure 7.6** demonstrates the progressive reduction in voltage following RF delivery at the mitral isthmus.

Mitral isthmus line ablation during sinus rhythm

Conduction gaps on the mitral isthmus are most often found near to the LAA and LIPV. This is probably related to the local anatomy and the difficulty inherent in maintaining a stable catheter position at this site. **Figure 7.7** shows EGMs recorded during proximal CS pacing at sites of conduction gaps in the mitral isthmus line:

- **Figure 7.7a** demonstrates a gap potential near the LIPV on distal pole recording (RFd), and slow conduction from the pacing site (CS 3–4) to CS 1–2 (star).

- **Figure 7.7b** shows very rapid conduction from the site of CS pacing to the distal CS recording site (RFd, arrow). This was recorded following extensive endocardial ablation at the mitral isthmus and is suggestive of an epicardial gap site.

- **Figure 7.7c** shows a gap potential at the ventricular aspect of the mitral isthmus. The gap potential is characterized by high-frequency, fractionated activity spanning approximately 80 ms. The insets show the catheter positions for each respective recorded EGM.

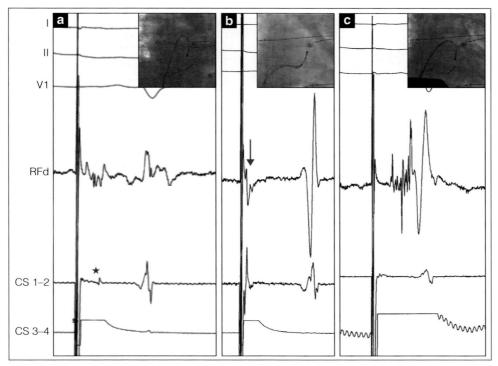

Figure 7.7. Mitral isthmus line ablation during sinus rhythm. CS: coronary sinus; d: distal; RF: ablation catheter.

Assessment of mitral isthmus line block

The principles for assessing conduction block across the roof line and CTI line apply equally to the mitral isthmus line. Assessment of conduction block should be performed as close to the line as possible, ie, the pacing and sensing catheters should ideally be placed either side of the line and adjacent to it.

During pacing, activation will spread centrifugally from the pacing site. If the pacing site is adjacent to the line, and the line is blocked, activation will spread away from the line, provided that there is no far-field capture of tissue on the other side of the line.

Figure 7.8 shows anteroposterior radiographs of the heart with a circumferential mapping catheter in the RAA, an irrigated ablation catheter at the base of the LAA lateral to the site of the ablated mitral isthmus linear lesion, and a deflectable decapolar catheter in the CS. The dashed lines indicate zones of conduction block. In **Figure 7.8a**, the pacing site is the distal bipole of the ablation catheter. In this situation, the activation fronts (white arrows) cannot traverse the line of conduction block at the mitral isthmus and cannot reach the posterior LA between or around the left PVs as this is the site of previous *en bloc* PV isolation. Therefore, activation proceeds from the pacing site, up the lateral wall of the LA, and across the roof, and activates the posterior wall in a craniocaudal direction, thereby activating the CS from proximal to distal. The delay is measured from the pacing stimulus to the EGM recorded at site 2, with activation at site 1 preceding site 2.

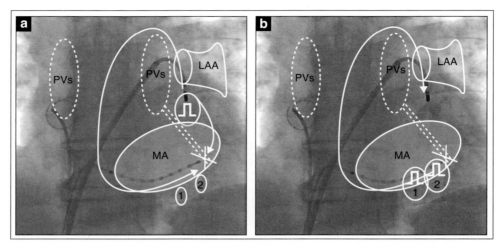

Figure 7.8. Assessment of mitral isthmus line block. LAA: left atrial appendage; MA: mitral annulus; PV: pulmonary vein.

In **Figure 7.8b**, the pacing site is switched to the distal CS bipole (site 2), and activation proceeds in the reverse direction to that shown in **Figure 7.8a**. By pacing from a more proximal position in the CS (site 1), the distance traveled by the wave front to achieve the lateral aspect of the line is shorter and, therefore, so is the measured delay.

In **Figure 7.9**, the tracings illustrate the electrographic assessment of mitral isthmus line block as described in **Figure 7.8**.

Figure 7.9a shows the recorded EGMs at the LAA and within the CS during pacing at the CS 3–4 bipole (equivalent to position 1 in **Figure 7.8**) when the CS 1–2 bipole is positioned immediately septal to the mitral isthmus line (equivalent to position 2 in **Figure 7.8**). The recorded delay to the lateral aspect of the line (RF catheter within the LAA) is 192 ms. When the pacing site is switched to the distal CS, the delay is longer (210 ms, **Figure 7.9b**), confirming the presence of septal-to-lateral conduction block. Widely separated local double potentials along the length of the ablation line are often observed (**Figure 7.9b**, arrow) during CS pacing. Bidirectional block is demonstrated in **Figure 7.9c** by pacing at the LAA. Activation of the CS proceeds from proximal to distal (arrow), with the longest delay recorded immediately adjacent to the line (CS 1–2).

Assessment of combined mitral isthmus block and roof-line block

When complete linear lesions have been created at both the mitral isthmus and the roof, assessment of the lesions is merely an extension of what has already been described for the individual lines.

With conduction block at the roof line (bold dashed line, **Figure 7.10a**), pacing of the LAA results in activation across the anterior aspect of the LA roof, down the septum across the floor of the LA, and simultaneous caudocranial activation of the posterior LA (site 1 earlier than sites 2 or 3).

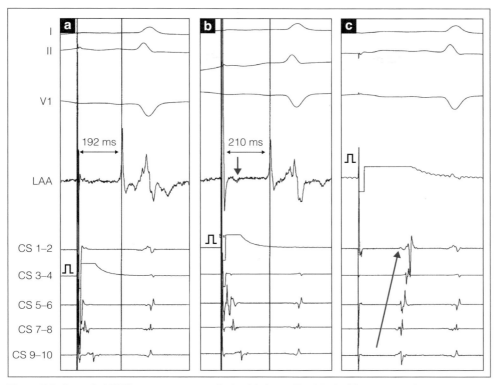

Figure 7.9. Recorded EGMs on assessment of mitral isthmus line block. CS: coronary sinus; LAA: left atrial appendage.

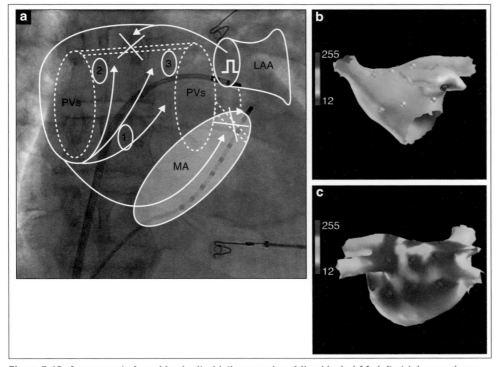

Figure 7.10. Assessment of combined mitral isthmus and roof-line block. LAA: left atrial appendage; MA: mitral annulus; PV: pulmonary vein.

In this setting, activation of the posterior LA should be earlier near the right PVs (site 2) than at the left PVs (site 3) provided that the mitral isthmus line is also blocked. The CS will be activated from proximal to distal.

Therefore, by demonstrating activation earlier on the right side of the posterior LA than on the left side, and a proximal-to-distal activation sequence within the CS, it is possible to conclude that both lines are blocked when pacing is performed from the LAA.

On **Figures 7.10b** and **c**, activation visualized on an imported LA geometry ElectroView map (Bard Electrophysiology, C R Bard, Inc, Lowell, MA, USA) illustrates the activation wave front circulating from low to high and right to left on the posterior wall (**Figure 7.10c**) during LAA pacing (anteroposterior view, **Figure 7.10a**).

Cavotricuspid isthmus ablation during atrial fibrillation

Ablation at the CTI is performed in all patients in our laboratory, regardless of whether the RA is the driving chamber for AF.

Figure 7.11a shows complex activity recorded on the ablation catheter at the CTI. With increasing ablation, local voltage is attenuated (**Figures 7.11b** and **c**). Once sinus rhythm has been restored, conduction block across the CTI can be assessed.

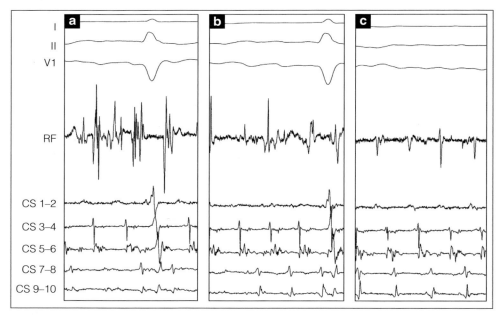

Figure 7.11. Ablation at the cavotricuspid isthmus during atrial fibrillation. CS: coronary sinus; RF: ablation catheter.

Cavotricuspid isthmus block assessment

Conduction block at the CTI is assessed using the principles of differential pacing. **Figure 7.12a** shows the radiographic position (inset) of the RF catheter on the ablation line during CS proximal pacing. A double potential is recorded, representing activity from both sides of the line, with the greatest delay measured at 140 ms. **Figure 7.12b** shows a shorter delay (118 ms) when the recording catheter is moved lateral to the line to the position shown in the radiographic inset. Note the change in P-wave morphology at the inferior leads (**Figure 7.12c**, arrow) during CS pacing when conduction block is achieved. The second component becomes more positive when lateral RA activation proceeds entirely in a craniocaudal direction.

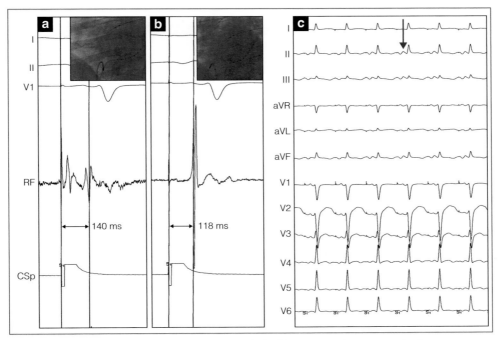

Figure 7.12. Assessment of cavotricuspid isthmus block. CS: coronary sinus; p: proximal; RF: ablation catheter.

8 | Atrial tachycardias in the context of atrial fibrillation ablation

Atrial tachycardia is seen in many patients during the index procedure for ablation of chronic atrial fibrillation and is the dominant mode of arrhythmia recurrence in patients in whom atrial fibrillation termination is achieved during the index procedure. This chapter describes an approach to diagnosis and treatment of atrial tachycardias seen in the context of atrial fibrillation ablation.

- Atrial tachycardia

- Macro re-entry

- Perimitral flutter

- Roof-dependent flutter

- Peritricuspid flutter

- Focal atrial tachycardia

- The importance of localized re-entry

- Localized re-entry near the roof line

- Focal point atrial tachycardia

- Practical approach

- Atrial tachycardia transition

- Difficult cases not solved by the algorithm

- Localized re-entry – the value of the post-pacing interval

- Perimitral macro re-entry with two gaps

Atrial tachycardia

Definitions

For the purposes of describing our approach to atrial tachycardias (ATs) arising in the context of catheter ablation of atrial fibrillation (AF), the following definitions are employed:

- *AT* is characterized by a monomorphic P-wave and a consistent intracardiac activation sequence.

- *Macro re-entry* is defined as a circuit involving more than three atrial segments (see Left atrial nomenclature, Chapter 1), that are usually >2 cm in diameter, and where >75% of the circuit is mapped.

- *Focal-point tachycardia* is defined as centrifugal activation originating from a discrete site, which incorporates automaticity, triggered activity, and re-entrant mechanisms where <75% of the cycle can be mapped in the chamber of interest.

- *Localized re-entry* constitutes a circuit involving one or two adjacent segments that are usually <2 cm in diameter, and span >75% of the cycle length (CL) within the involved segments.

As a general rule, macro re-entrant AT is easy to diagnose but is more difficult to treat, while focal AT is difficult to map but is easily ablated.

Figure 8.1 illustrates the three mechanisms of arrhythmogenesis found in patients with AT during and following previous AF ablation. **a** refers to counterclockwise macro re-entry

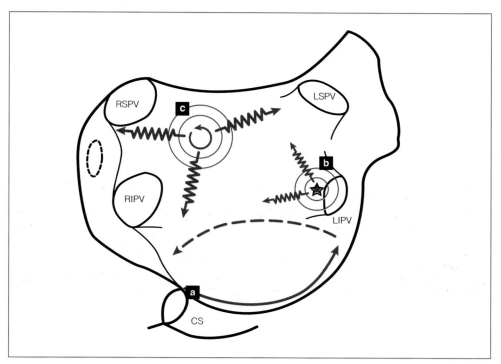

Figure 8.1. CS: coronary sinus; LIPV: left inferior pulmonary vein; LSPV: left superior pulmonary vein; RIPV: right inferior pulmonary vein; RSPV: right superior pulmonary vein.

around the mitral annulus (MA). **b** refers to a focal point tachycardia where activation can be mapped to a single discrete point (in this case the left inferior pulmonary vein [LIPV]), with centrifugal spread to the surrounding atrium. **c** refers to a localized re-entry in the posterior left atrium (LA) with centrifugal activation to the surrounding atrium.

Macro re-entry

Approximately 47% of ATs are macro re-entries. The most frequent are perimitral circuits (58%), followed by roof-dependent circuits (30%) and peritricuspid circuits (5%). The rest consist of more complex arrhythmias, including double-loop re-entry and circuits passing through a gap between the LIPV and left atrial appendage (LAA).

Typical activation wave fronts within the LA during macro re-entry are illustrated in **Figure 8.2** using a 3D segmentation of the LA in an anteroposterior view (EP Navigator, Philips, Eindhoven, The Netherlands). The directions of activation of the posterior and anterior walls are indicated by dashed arrows and solid arrows, respectively.

In the case of a perimitral circuit (**Figure 8.2a**), coronary sinus (CS) activation demonstrates a distal-to-proximal activation in 50% of cases and a proximal-to-distal activation in the remainder. In both clockwise and counterclockwise perimitral flutter, the LA is activated from the annulus towards the posterior part of the LA. Therefore, opposing positions on the MA cannot be activated simultaneously. This observation is useful in recognizing perimitral re-entry during the mapping phase.

In roof-dependent macro re-entry (**Figure 8.2b**), the CS is activated from proximal to distal position in 30%, consistent with a circuit around the right pulmonary veins (PVs), and from distal to proximal position in 30%, suggestive of a circuit around the left PVs. In 40% of cases, there is no preferential direction of activation of the CS, which may be as a result of slow conduction related to prior ablation. For a roof-dependent circuit, the LA is activated from the roof towards the annulus in either the anterior or posterior segment and in the reverse direction on the opposing LA segment. However, opposing surfaces cannot be activated simultaneously. Recognition of this is critical during the mapping of these circuits.

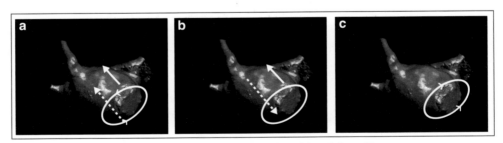

Figure 8.2. Macro re-entry: **(a)** perimitral; **(b)** roof dependent; **(c)** peritricuspid.

For a tachycardia around the tricuspid annulus (**Figure 8.2c**), the CS is activated from proximal to distal position, and both the anterior and posterior MA undergo near-simultaneous activation. The activation front is ascending in both anterior and posterior segments.

Perimitral flutter

Figure 8.3 illustrates a clockwise perimitral circuit. Activation spanning all of the CL can be followed throughout the MA (**Figures 8.3a–d**) using the radiofrequency energy (RF) catheter: lateral-to-septal activation at the CS and septal-to-lateral activation anteriorly. Both posterior (dashed arrow) and anterior (solid arrow) walls are activated in an ascending direction as demonstrated on the inset anteroposterior radiograph of the LA.

Entrainment at the anterior and posterior MA and on the mitral isthmus gave a post-pacing interval (PPI) of 10 ms. At the mitral isthmus (**Figure 8.3d**), a long, fractionated electrogram (EGM) corresponding to a gap potential was recorded (star). Ablation at this site broke the circuit and restored sinus rhythm (tachycardia termination) (**Figure 8.3e**).

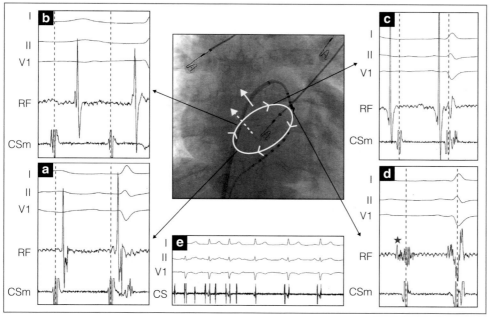

Figure 8.3. Perimitral flutter. The coronary sinus (CS) timing reference has been emphasized using red dashed lines. CSm: coronary sinus mid-portion; RF: ablation catheter.

Roof-dependent flutter

The tracing shown in **Figure 8.4** illustrates a roof-dependent circuit in the context of prior AF ablation, including an attempt to block the roof. There is ascending activation of the posterior wall (dashed arrow, from **Figure 8.4a** to **b**), while the anterior wall (solid arrow) is activated in a descending direction (from **Figure 8.4c** to **d**). The CS timing reference is emphasized using the dashed red lines.

On the roof, a potential spanning the rest of the CL is recorded, corresponding to the gap on the line (**Figure 8.4b**, star). RF application at this site restored sinus rhythm after a few seconds (**Figure 8.4e**). A double potential is recorded on the ablation site during sinus rhythm (**Figure 8.4e**, star). The second deflection corresponds to late activation of the posterior wall, suggesting roof-line block.

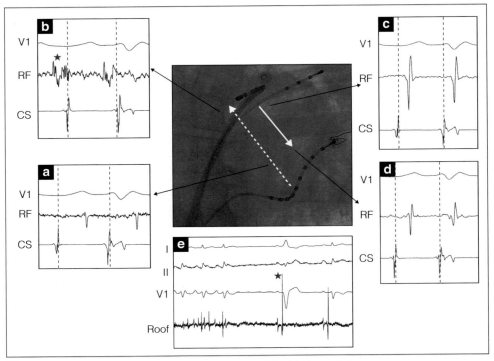

Figure 8.4. Roof-dependent flutter. CS: coronary sinus; RF: ablation catheter.

Peritricuspid flutter

The case shown in **Figure 8.5** illustrates a typical right atrial flutter (circular arrow) diagnosed after conversion from persistent AF. Activation in the LA was ascending both anteriorly (solid white arrow) and posteriorly (dashed white arrow). Activation of the CS occurred in a septal-to-lateral direction (lower curved white arrow), as well as at the anterior MA (upper curved white arrow).

All of the circuit was mapped around the tricuspid annulus with the distal CS as a timing reference (**Figures 8.5a–c**). Activity in mid cycle was recorded (panel **a**) at the 6 o'clock position on the tricuspid annulus, at the 1 o'clock position immediately before the reference (panel **b**), and at the 11 o'clock position immediately after the reference (panel **c**). Coronary sinus activation was from proximal to distal position (arrow, panel **a**).

Entrainment at the cavotricuspid isthmus (CTI) confirmed that it lay within the circuit. A linear lesion joining the tricuspid annulus and the inferior vena cava (IVC) restored sinus rhythm. The red vertical dashed lines emphasize the CS timing reference.

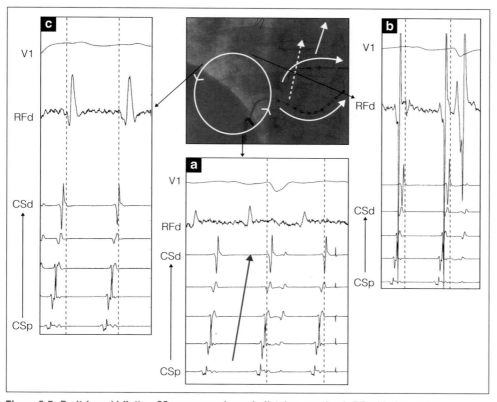

Figure 8.5. Peritricuspid flutter. CS: coronary sinus; d: distal; p: proximal; RF: ablation catheter.

Focal atrial tachycardia

Approximately 53% of ATs are focal. Among those, localized re-entries are the most frequent AT mechanism, representing 71% of focal ATs (and 37% of total ATs). The preferential regions for focal ATs are shown in **Figure 8.6**. These are the PV–LA junction, left septum, and entrance of the LAA.

Localization of focal AT is generally related to sites targeted during EGM-based AF ablation. Injury or edema of atrial tissue following RF application could represent the substrate for arrhythmia, acting as an anchor point capable of maintaining re-entry. Therefore, the mechanism of AT after AF ablation may be different from that of spontaneous AT.

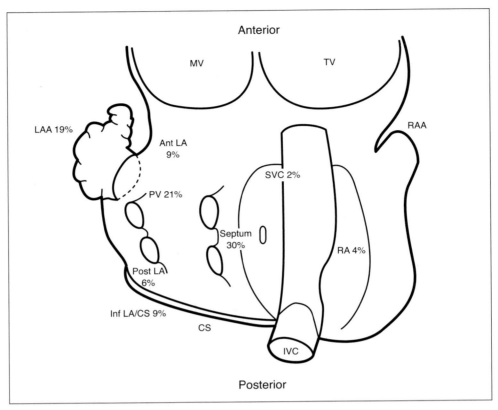

Figure 8.6. Preferential regions of focal atrial tachycardia (AT). Percentages indicate the relative contribution of each region to the total focal AT burden. Ant: anterior; CS: coronary sinus; Inf: inferior; IVC: inferior vena cava; LA: left atrium; LAA; left atrial appendage; MV: mitral valve; Post: posterior; PV: pulmonary vein; RA: right atrium; RAA: right atrial appendage; SVC: superior vena cava; TV: tricuspid valve.

The presence of pre-existing LA scarring (which may be idiopathic or related to underlying structural heart disease) may also result in local slow conduction areas predisposing to re-entry.

Mapping and ablation of AT is an indispensable step in the AF ablation process, and often represents the difference between procedural success and failure.

The importance of localized re-entry

While the earliest diastolic potentials are tracked during mapping for focal point AT, local activity spanning all of the CL has to be documented in the context of localized re-entry. If just a limited part of the CL can be mapped in the suspected region of origin, a re-entrant mechanism is excluded. If local activity spans most or all of the atrial tachycardia cycle length (ATCL) (ie, >70%), it suggests a re-entrant mechanism.

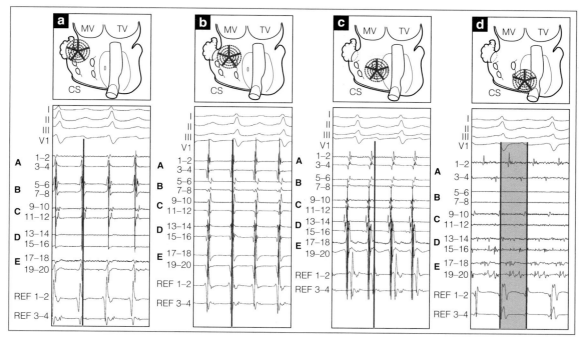

Figure 8.7. Localized re-entry. The upper panels show the anatomic position as the catheter is moved from the lateral to septal position; the lower panels show the electrical recordings at those sites. CS: coronary sinus; MV: mitral valve; REF: reference catheter; TV: tricuspid valve.

Approximately half of patients harboring localized re-entry can have their arrhythmia induced by programmed stimulation, and the re-entrant mechanism can be confirmed by entrainment maneuvers.

The tracings in **Figure 8.7** illustrate localized activation spreading centrifugally from an area of <2 cm in diameter. By moving the 20-pole catheter in the posterior wall from lateral-to-septal (from **Figures 8.7a–c**), organized local activity was earlier compared with a CS reference (red line), consistent with centrifugal activation from the septum. In the septum, local activity spanned all of the CL (**Figure 8.7d**, pink-shaded bar), which suggested re-entry.

Mapping of a localized re-entry may also be performed with a conventional RF catheter and a fixed timing reference to permit exploration of the tachycardia window of interest, (ie, the CL), as represented by the pink-shaded bars in **Figure 8.8**. These tracings illustrate a localized re-entry spreading out centrifugally from the posterior LA.

Mapping of three different but closely adjacent anatomical spots (**Figures 8.8a–c**) within an area of <2 cm in the high posterior LA showed local activity (within the red dashed lines) spanning the entire CL (pink-shaded bars). The ablation catheter was then placed in the center of this region (**Figure 8.8d**), and recorded a very-low-voltage signal (0.04 mV) spanning all of the CL. RF application at this point restored sinus rhythm after a few seconds.

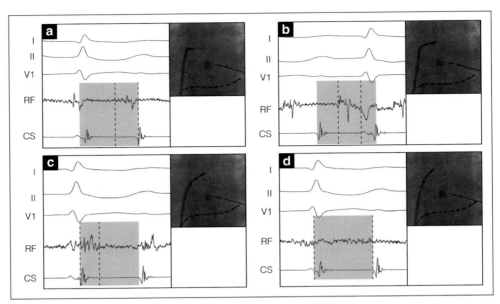

Figure 8.8. Localized re-entry. CS: coronary sinus; RF: ablation catheter.

A challenging situation is encountered when a focal arrhythmia is located in the vicinity of a complete ablation line. This is relatively frequent in the context of persistent AF ablation.

The activation front will propagate all around the atrium, simulating the activation observed during a macro re-entry through a gap in the ablation line.

The case shown in **Figure 8.9** illustrates a focal tachycardia located posterior to a complete mitral isthmus line. The LA activation is compatible with a clockwise perimitral macro re-entry (**Figures 8.9a–d**). However, at least one third of the cycle could not be accounted for (**Figures 8.9c** and **d**), which should not be the case with perimitral re-entry. Furthermore, entrainment maneuvers displayed a very long PPI in the anterior LA, while posterior entrainment gave a PPI within 30 ms of the ATCL. Mapping of the area posterior to the mitral isthmus line revealed very-low-voltage local activity spanning much of the CL (**Figure 8.9e**, pink-shaded bar). The blocked mitral isthmus line is shown as a serration joining the posterolateral mitral valve annulus to the left inferior pulmonary vein (LIPV), and the star indicates the site of origin of the localized re-entry circuit. The timing reference points at the beginning of each cycle of the tachycardia are indicated by the dashed red lines either side of the pink-shaded bar. These align with the CS reference. Ablation of this localized re-entry was subsequently performed, with restoration of sinus rhythm.

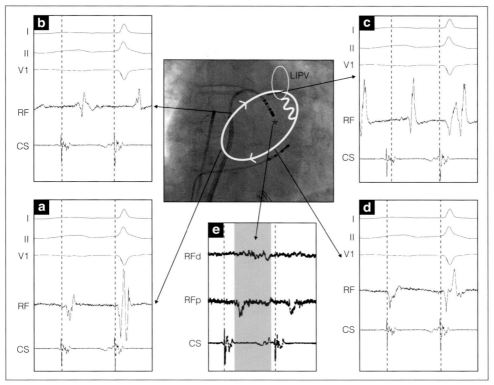

Figure 8.9. Localized re-rentry near the mitral isthmus. CS: coronary sinus; d: distal; LIPV: left inferior pulmonary vein; p: proximal; RF: ablation catheter.

Localized re-entry near the roof line

The case shown in **Figure 8.10** illustrates localized re-entry originating from the posterior wall, with a previous roof line. The activation front was consistent with a roof-dependent macro re-entry (**Figures 8.10a–d**), ascending the anterior wall (**Figures 8.10a–b**, solid white arrow) and descending the posterior wall (**Figures 8.10c–d**, dashed white arrow). The mapped activity spanned the entire CL (marked by the dashed red vertical lines), but slow conduction was present in the anteroseptal area (**Figure 8.10a**), resulting in a misleading diagnosis.

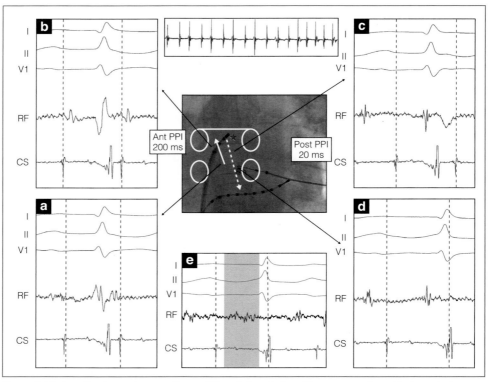

Figure 8.10. Localized re-entry near the roof line. Ant: anterior; CS: coronary sinus; Post: posterior; PPI: post-pacing interval; RF: ablation catheter.

Irregularity constituted >15% of the CL (inset electrocardiogram [ECG]) and the anterior PPI was very long (+200 ms), which was suggestive more of a focus originating from the high posterior LA. Mapping of this area in the high posterior LA, close to the roof line, revealed very-low-voltage local activity spanning most of the CL (**Figure 8.10e**, pink-shaded bar). Ablation at this site (indicated by the star) terminated tachycardia.

Focal point atrial tachycardia

Focal-point AT represents 29% of focal ATs. Most cases originate from the PVs and their ostia. The tracing shown in **Figure 8.11** illustrates a focal-point tachycardia mapped in the region of the left PV ostia with a 20-pole catheter (inset). All of the spines display a proximal-to-distal pattern (arrows), with the earliest potential recorded on the proximal bipoles of spines A and E (stars).

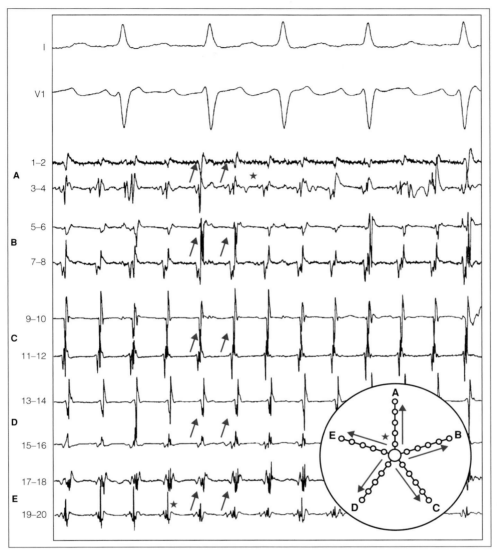

Figure 8.11. Focal point atrial tachycardia.

The inset catheter schematic depicts the focal-point site and the resultant activation sequence of the multipolar catheter from proximal to distal positions on all spines.

Practical approach

The principles previously described for mapping of AT have been incorporated into a diagnostic algorithm (**Figure 8.12**), and are listed here:

- Confirmation of PV isolation.

- ATCL variability (CL variability is calculated by dividing the CL range by the mean CL averaged over 30 cycles):

  – If >15%, suggestive of focal AT

  – If <15%, no discriminating value

- Macro re-entry: activation mapping to assess the likelihood of perimitral, roof-dependent, or peritricuspid circuit. Entrainment maneuvers are used to confirm the diagnosis.

- Non-macro re-entrant AT: track the earliest area. Entrainment maneuvers are used to evaluate the site of origin.

  – Localized re-entry: look for long-duration fractionated potentials spanning most or all of the CL

  – Others: target the earliest activity

- Nonconsistent: more complex tachycardia, change in AT, or redo mapping.

Prospective evaluation of this algorithm leads to the diagnosis and successful treatment of AT in the vast majority of cases.

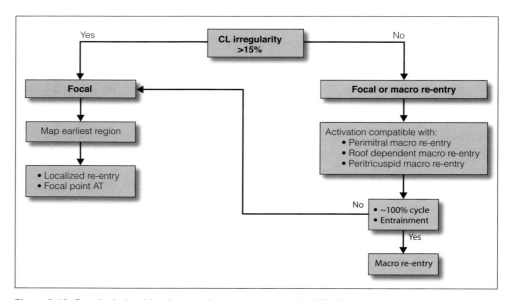

Figure 8.12. Practical algorithm for mapping atrial tachycardia (AT). CL: cycle length.

Atrial tachycardia transition

It is crucial to remain watchful to identify any change in CL and/or activation that indicates that ablation has modified the arrhythmia. Any transition to another tachycardia requires a repeat assessment using the practical algorithm to define the mechanism. The transition may be obvious or almost imperceptible, as shown in **Figure 8.13** by the subtle change in CL.

Although unusual, it is possible that a tachycardia can be successfully terminated without any change in CL or activation as shown by the CS reference catheter. A change in global atrial activation will only be apparent by remapping the chamber and analyzing the surface P-wave morphology closely. This justifies repeating entrainment maneuvers in the presence of a resistant tachycardia to be sure that it has not changed to another one, or that an error has not been made in the initial mapping of the AT.

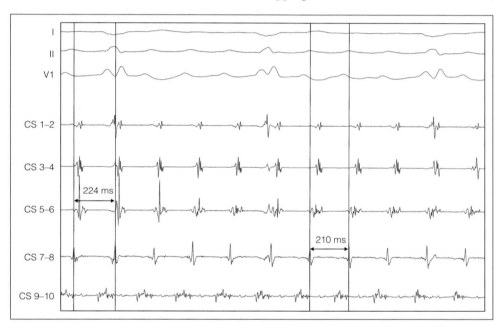

Figure 8.13. Atrial tachycardia transition. CS: coronary sinus.

Difficult cases not solved by the algorithm

In the case of extensive scarring or ablation, mapping of AT can be challenging with the practical algorithm (**Figure 8.14**). In this situation, three methods can be used to facilitate identification and ablation of the AT:

Entrainment maneuvers performed during the arrhythmia will point towards a focal origin by demonstrating long-return CLs around the MA, roof line, or tricuspid annulus, except at sites adjacent to the focus (by definition, less than two segments).

For localized re-entry, local activity spanning all of the ATCL can be demonstrated at an area of earliest activity.

For focal point AT, an area of early activity may exhibit mid-diastolic potentials.

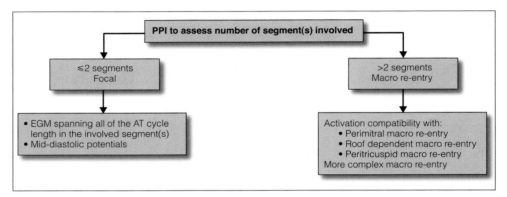

Figure 8.14. Difficult cases algorithm. AT: atrial tachycardia; EGM: electrogram; PPI: post-pacing interval.

Localized re-entry – the value of the post-pacing interval

The tracings shown in **Figure 8.15** illustrate a case with prior extensive LA ablation to convert AF, including the left mitral isthmus line.

Conduction around the MA was compatible with a perimitral circuit (lateral to septal anteriorly and septal to lateral posteriorly). The PPI was <30 ms at the anterior annulus, but >30 ms at the CS. This made a macro re-entrant perimitral circuit unlikely and suggested a focal AT lateral to a completed left mitral isthmus line. Mapping was performed in this area, where a site displaying most of the CL was found at the anterior mouth of the LAA. However, the PPI was +100 ms at this site (**Figure 8.15a**).

Another site displaying most of the CL with a gradient-of-activation EGM pattern and a short PPI (+10 ms) was mapped to the anterior LA (**Figure 8.15b**). Ablation at this site restored sinus rhythm, and a local double potential was visualized after ablation (**Figure 8.15c**, arrows) in sinus rhythm.

This case illustrates how useful the PPI can be in difficult cases. During entrainment, attention must be paid to avoid induction of AF at short CLs, or the possibility of conversion to another AT.

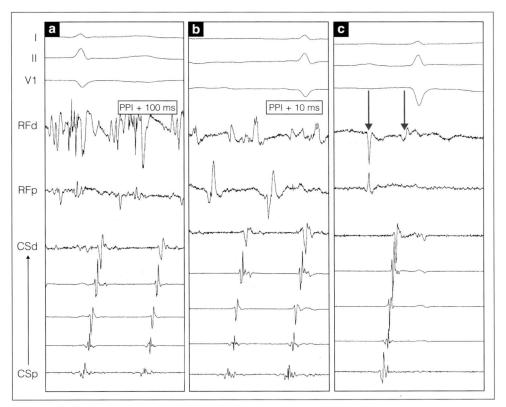

Figure 8.15. Localized re-entry. CS: coronary sinus; d: distal; p: proximal; RF: ablation catheter.

Perimitral macro re-entry with two gaps

In the patient described in **Figure 8.16**, following ablation at a site of fractionation at the LA roof consistent with a conduction gap, there was a dramatic change in P-wave morphology and an AT emerged with regular alternation of CL between 266 and 364 ms (**Figure 8.16a**), and proximal-to-distal activation within the CS.

Electroanatomic mapping (CARTO, Biosense Webster, Inc, Diamond Bar, CA, USA) was performed in which the window of interest of the more rapid tachycardia (266 ms) was explored; an activation sequence consistent with a counterclockwise perimitral flutter was obtained (**Figure 8.16b**). Subsequently, a second electroanatomic map was constructed for the longer CL tachycardia (364 ms). Again, the entire CL could be mapped around the MA (**Figure 8.16c**).

Following termination of the AT by pacing, the roof line was confirmed as intact. Two discrete gap sites on the previously ablated mitral isthmus were mapped and ablated to restore conduction block across this line.

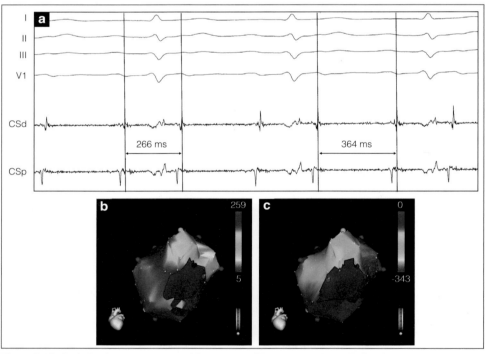

Figure 8.16. Perimitral macro re-entry with two gaps. CS: coronary sinus; d: distal; p: proximal.

9 | Electromechanical consequences of ablation

This chapter describes some unusual examples of disturbed intra-atrial conduction which can occur in the context of catheter ablation for persistent atrial fibrillation.

- Consequences of ablation

- Atrial arrhythmia confined within the coronary sinus

- Delayed left atrial appendage activity

- Late fractionated potential in sinus rhythm

- Left atrial appendage disconnection

- Left atrial appendage as an arrhythmogenic source

Consequences of ablation

Electrophysiological phenomena that are otherwise vanishingly rare are commonly seen as a result of catheter ablation of persistent atrial fibrillation (AF). These may include dissociation or electrical disconnection of the left atrial appendage (LAA) and coronary sinus (CS). Remarkable local delays in activation can also be seen.

A voltage mapping study of 40 patients at >1 month after ablation showed areas of scarring and low voltage accounting for approximately 30% each of the total left atrial (LA) surface area (Takahashi et al, 2007; *see* Bibliography). The area of scarring outside of the pulmonary vein (PV) region represented between 8% and 14% of the LA surface area. In this study, LA contraction was restored in all patients in sinus rhythm at follow-up.

Figure 9.1 shows an electroanatomic LA voltage map (CARTO) performed 3 months following ablation for persistent AF (**Figures 9.1a–c,** biatrial map **Figure 9.1d**). A low voltage cut-off of 0.5 mV was chosen: voltages of >0.5 mV are represented in pink; those of <0.5 mV are represented by other colors. Note that the low-voltage areas were confined to the PVs, roof, septum, inferior LA, and mitral isthmus. Grey represents atrial scarring (voltage of <0.05 mV).

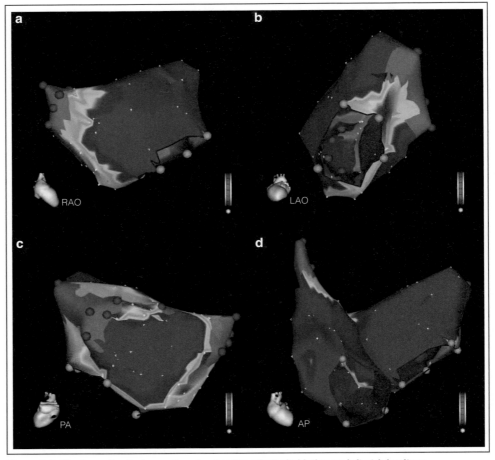

Figure 9.1. Electroanatomical mapping showing the effect of ablation on left atrial voltage.
AP: anteroposterior; LAO: left anterior oblique; PA: posteroanterior; RAO: right anterior oblique.

Atrial arrhythmia confined within the coronary sinus

The aim of CS ablation is not to isolate this structure. However, isolation is occasionally necessary when this vessel is mapped as a centrifugal source of activation driving AF but the exact site of origin cannot be accurately determined.

In the case shown in **Figure 9.2**, isolation of the CS was accomplished by longitudinal endocardial and epicardial ablation, followed by circumferential ablation at the CS ostium. This resulted in restoration of sinus rhythm followed by bursts of variable cycle length (CL) rapid activity (150–230 ms; **Figure 9.2a**, star) confined within the CS. Only 35% of the CL could be mapped.

Ablation targeting the earliest activity (mid CS) terminated this arrhythmia 20 minutes after CS dissociation, after which a much slower dissociated rhythm in the CS was observed (**Figure 9.2b**, stars). AF could not be induced by burst pacing from three sites within the CS.

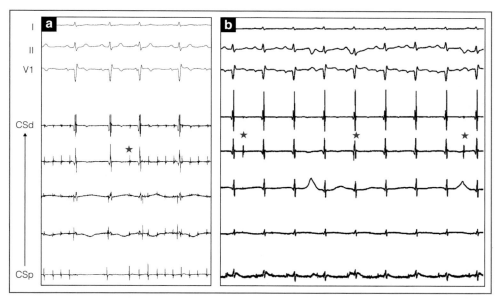

Figure 9.2. Atrial arrhythmia confined within the coronary sinus (CS). d: distal; p: proximal.

Delayed left atrial appendage activity

Conduction into the LAA may be markedly affected in the setting of pre-existing spontaneous local scarring, extensive circumferential ablation at the LAA mouth, or the combined effect of lesion extension from the left PVs, mitral isthmus, and anterior LA.

Figure 9.3 shows the impact of extensive ablation in the region of the LAA. Greatly delayed LAA depolarization is recorded within this structure (stars). This corresponds to a small wave on the electrocardiogram (ECG) that appears after the QRS complex (arrows).

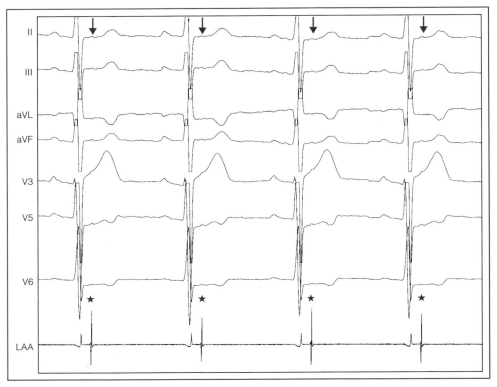

Figure 9.3. Delayed left atrial appendage (LAA) activity.

Late fractionated potential in sinus rhythm

Late atrial activation, after the QRS complex, is recorded by the RF catheter positioned on the posterior ridge of the LAA. The first beat on the tracing shown in **Figure 9.4** is a sinus beat. Note the fractionated character of the local recordings, indicative of slow conduction into the posterior ridge of the LAA resulting from prior ablation.

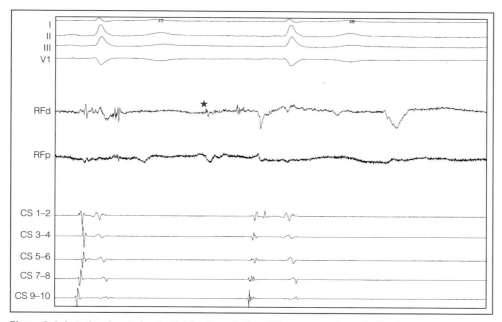

Figure 9.4. Late fractionated potential in sinus rhythm. CS: coronary sinus; d: distal; p: proximal; RF: ablation catheter.

The second beat is a premature atrial beat. The precocity of the local electrograms (EGMs) recorded by the radiofrequency energy (RF) catheter relative to the CS indicates the local origin of the activity (star). The long duration of the low-amplitude, fractionated EGMs indicates slow conduction away from this region and its potential role as an arrhythmogenic substrate. This potential may represent the last route of conduction to the LAA and, although possibly arrhythmogenic, the risk of ablating this site must be weighed against the risk of electrical disconnection of this structure and lifelong anticoagulation.

Left atrial appendage disconnection

The case illustrated in **Figure 9.5** describes the impact of extensive ablation of the segments surrounding the LAA in a patient with persistent AF of 17 months' duration.

Figure 9.5a shows an atrial tachycardia (AT) originating in the LAA with 2:1 conduction to the atria as indicated by the arrows (conduction) and lines (conduction block). Note that the P-wave morphology and axis are not consistent with sinus rhythm. Further attempts to ablate this focal arrhythmia (stars) resulted in inadvertent disconnection of the LAA (**Figure 9.5b**), apparent by restoration of sinus rhythm (note the different P-wave morphology compared with **Figure 9.5a**) and no relationship with the ongoing AT confined to the LAA (exit block). After further ablation, the AT terminated. Dissociated automatic activity (**Figure 9.5c**; open star) was recorded within the LAA, also indicating exit block.

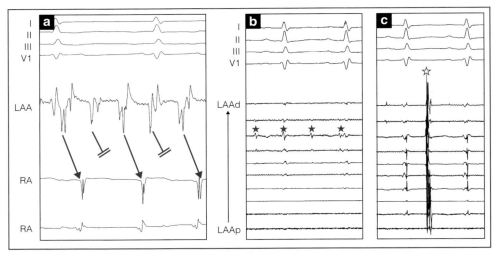

Figure 9.5. Left atrial appendage (LAA) disconnection. d: distal; p: proximal; RA: right atrium.

Left atrial appendage as an arrhythmogenic source

In **Figure 9.6**, two consecutive phenomena can be seen following extensive LA ablation. These emphasize the arrhythmogenicity of this structure:

- Slow dissociated LAA activity (stars) occurring during sinus rhythm.

- A rapid burst of activity from within the LAA without conduction to the LA.

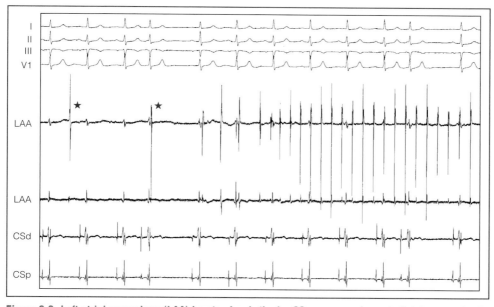

Figure 9.6. Left atrial appendage (LAA) bursts of arrhythmia. CS: coronary sinus; d: distal; p: proximal.

10 | Ablation of persistent atrial fibrillation: from start to finish

This chapter describes a typical real life case of persistent atrial fibrillation and takes the reader step by step through the process of terminating atrial fibrillation, mapping intermediate atrial tachycardias, and finally, restoring sinus rhythm.

- Case description

- Progressive increase in atrial fibrillation cycle length

- Conversion to atrial tachycardia

- Mapping and ablation of atrial tachycardias

- Restoration of sinus rhythm

Case description

The patient is a 55-year-old physical education instructor with idiopathic dilated cardiomyopathy (left ventricular ejection fraction of 0.35), and atrial fibrillation (AF) for 2 years, persistent for 15 months. The left atrium (LA) was greatly dilated, with a diameter of 60 mm in the parasternal short-axis echocardiographic view.

Following an unsuccessful electrical cardioversion 1 year previously, amiodarone was discontinued because of hyperthyroidism. Atrial fibrillation cycle length (AFCL) was calculated before the hospitalization using the V1 electrocardiogram (ECG) lead (163 ms), and just before ablation in the right atrial appendage (RAA; 164 ms) and in the left atrial appendage (LAA; 171 ms) (**Figure 10.1**). This indicated an approximately 95% likelihood of restoring normal sinus rhythm.

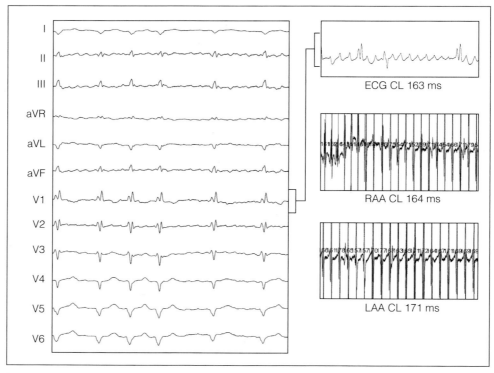

Figure 10.1. Case report: 12-lead electrocardiogram (ECG) showing baseline atrial fibrillation cycle length (CL). LAA: left atrial appendage; RAA: right atrial appendage.

Progressive increase in atrial fibrillation cycle length

Isolation of the pulmonary veins (PVs) resulted in an increase in the AFCL to 185 ms in the LAA (+14 ms) and to 178 ms in the RAA (+14 ms, **Figure 10.2a**). Linear ablation along the LA roof had no impact on the AFCL (**Figure 10.2b**). Subsequent ablation at the septum, posterior LA, and inferior LA prolonged the AFCL to 190 ms in both chambers, with pauses demonstrated in the coronary sinus (CS) (**Figure 10.2c**, star) and reflected in the RAA.

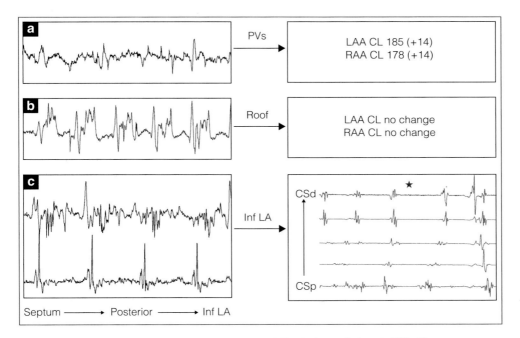

Figure 10.2. Case report: progressive increase in atrial fibrillation cycle length (CL). CS: coronary sinus; d: distal; Inf LA: inferior left atrium; LAA: left atrial appendage; p: proximal; PV: pulmonary vein; RAA: right atrial appendage.

Conversion to atrial tachycardia

The pauses in CS and RAA activity during inferior LA ablation at sites of continuous activity suggested an important role for this region in the perpetuation of AF. Ablation focused at the inferior LA resulted in termination of AF by conversion to atrial tachycardia (AT) (**Figure 10.3**, star).

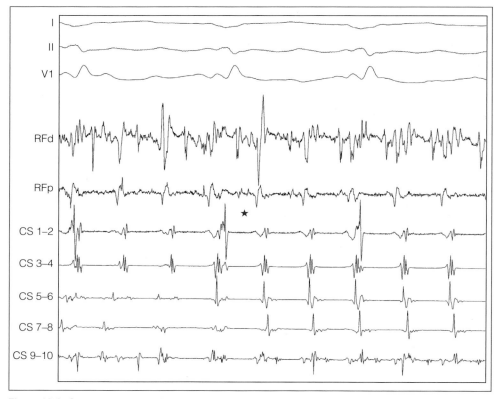

Figure 10.3. Case report: conversion to atrial tachycardia. CS: coronary sinus; d: distal; p: proximal; RF: ablation catheter.

Mapping and ablation of atrial tachycardias

The first AT (**Figure 10.4**, AT1) was progressively mapped to the inferior LA, from where centrifugal activation emanated, and local electrograms (EGMs) spanned the majority of the ATCL (194 ms). Ablation there at the inferior LA resulted in conversion to AT2, which displayed a longer ATCL (210 ms). AT2 also displayed the properties of a localized re-entry active at the CS ostium (centrifugal activation from this area with local activity spanning most of the cycle length [CL]). Ablation at the CS ostium converted the rhythm to AT3 (276 ms).

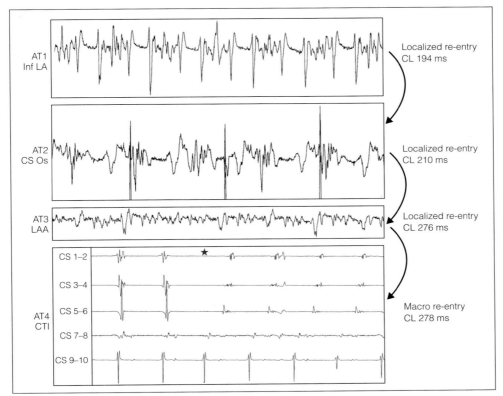

Figure 10.4. Case report: mapping and ablation of atrial tachycardias (ATs). CL: cycle length; CS Os: coronary sinus ostium; CTI: cavotricuspid isthmus; Inf LA: inferior left atrium; LAA: left atrial appendage.

AT3 was similarly mapped to a centrifugal site on the posterior ridge of the LAA, where low-voltage activity covering most of the CL was again visible. Ablation here terminated this tachycardia and converted the patient to AT4 (278 ms, star). AT4 was identified as typical right atrial flutter by mapping the tricuspid annulus. The transition from AT3 to AT4 without a change in CL suggests three diagnostic possibilities:

- AT4 is entrained by AT3 and revealed only when AT3 is terminated.

- AT4 is the underlying tachycardia mechanism, and the change in intracardiac activation is secondary to the ablation performed at the base of the LAA when treating AT3.

- AT3 and AT4 are independent, but simultaneous, tachycardias of the same CL.

Only real-time mapping of the intracardiac activation sequence allowed us to form a conclusion, which was that AT4 was entrained by AT3.

Restoration of sinus rhythm

Ablation in the cavotricuspid isthmus (CTI) resulted in termination of AT4. After a nearly 9-second pause (requiring pacing), a narrow-complex escape rhythm was followed shortly afterwards by spontaneous sinus rhythm (**Figure 10.5**).

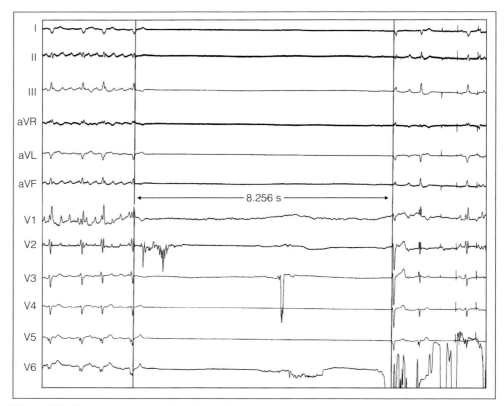

Figure 10.5. Case report: restoration of sinus rhythm.

Bibliography

The reference list is not intended to be exhaustive and should direct the interested reader to a more detailed exploration of some of the concepts described in this book, in addition to fundamental contributions from other world-renowned groups in this field.

Cappato R, Calkins H, Chen SA, et al. Worldwide survey on the methods, efficacy, and safety of catheter ablation for human atrial fibrillation. *Circulation* 2005;111:1100–5.

Cosio FG, Palacios J, Vidal JM, et al. Electrophysiologic studies in atrial fibrillation. Slow conduction of premature impulses: a possible manifestation of the background for reentry. *Am J Cardiol* 1983;51:122–30.

Haissaguerre M, Jais P, Shah DC, et al. Spontaneous initiation of atrial fibrillation by ectopic beats originating in the pulmonary veins. *N Engl J Med* 1998;339:659–66.

Haissaguerre M, Shah DC, Jais P, et al. Electrophysiological breakthroughs from the left atrium to the pulmonary veins. *Circulation* 2000;102:2463–5.

Haissaguerre M, Sanders P, Hocini M, et al. Changes in atrial fibrillation cycle length and inducibility during catheter ablation and their relation to outcome. *Circulation* 2004;109:3007–13.

Haissaguerre M, Hocini M, Sanders P, et al. Catheter ablation of long-lasting persistent atrial fibrillation: clinical outcome and mechanisms of subsequent arrhythmias. *J Cardiovasc Electrophysiol* 2005;16:1138–47.

Haissaguerre M, Sanders P, Hocini M, et al. Catheter ablation of long-lasting persistent atrial fibrillation: critical structures for termination. *J Cardiovasc Electrophysiol* 2005;16:1125–37.

Haissaguerre M, Hocini M, Sanders P, et al. Localized sources maintaining atrial fibrillation organized by prior ablation. *Circulation* 2006;113:616–25.

Haissaguerre M, Hocini M, Takahashi Y, et al. Impact of catheter ablation of the coronary sinus on paroxysmal or persistent atrial fibrillation. *J Cardiovasc Electrophysiol* 2007;18:378–86.

Haissaguerre M, Lim KT, Jacquemet V, et al. Atrial fibrillatory cycle length: computer simulation and potential clinical significance. *Europace* 2007;9(Suppl. 6):64–70.

Hocini M, Jais P, Sanders P, et al. Techniques, evaluation, and consequences of linear block at the left atrial roof in paroxysmal atrial fibrillation: a prospective randomized study. *Circulation* 2005;112:3688–96.

Hsu LF, Jais P, Sanders P, et al. Catheter ablation for atrial fibrillation in congestive heart failure. *N Engl J Med* 2004;351:2373–83.

Jais P, Haissaguerre M, Shah D, et al. Regional disparities of endocardial atrial activation in paroxysmal atrial fibrillation. *Pacing Clin Electrophysiol* 1996;19:1998–2003.

Jais P, Hocini M, Hsu LF, et al. Technique and results of linear ablation at the mitral isthmus. *Circulation* 2004;110:2996–3002.

Kalifa J, Tanaka K, Zaitsev AV, et al. Mechanisms of wave fractionation at boundaries of high-frequency excitation in the posterior left atrium of the isolated sheep heart during atrial fibrillation. *Circulation* 2006;113:626–33.

Lazar S, Dixit S, Marchlinski FE, et al. Presence of left-to-right atrial frequency gradient in paroxysmal but not persistent atrial fibrillation in humans. *Circulation* 2004;110:3181–6.

Lin WS, Tai CT, Hsieh MH, et al. Catheter ablation of paroxysmal atrial fibrillation initiated by non-pulmonary vein ectopy. *Circulation* 2003;107:3176–83.

Markides V, Schilling RJ, Ho SY, et al. Characterization of left atrial activation in the intact human heart. *Circulation* 2003;107:733–9.

Morillo CA, Klein GJ, Jones DL, et al. Chronic rapid atrial pacing. Structural, functional, and electrophysiological characteristics of a new model of sustained atrial fibrillation. *Circulation* 1995;91:1588–95.

Nademanee K, McKenzie J, Kosar E, et al. A new approach for catheter ablation of atrial fibrillation: mapping of the electrophysiologic substrate. *J Am Coll Cardiol* 2004;43:2044–53.

Oral H, Pappone C, Chugh A, et al. Circumferential pulmonary-vein ablation for chronic atrial fibrillation. *N Engl J Med* 2006;354:934–41.

Ouyang F, Ernst S, Chun J, et al. Electrophysiological findings during ablation of persistent atrial fibrillation with electroanatomic mapping and double LASSO catheter technique. *Circulation* 2005;112:3038–48.

Pappone C, Rosanio S, Oreto G, et al. Circumferential radiofrequency ablation of pulmonary vein ostia: a new anatomic approach for curing atrial fibrillation. *Circulation* 2000;102:2619–28.

Rostock T, Rotter M, Sanders P, et al. High-density activation mapping of fractionated electrograms in the atria of patients with paroxysmal atrial fibrillation. *Heart Rhythm* 2006;3:27–34.

Sanders P, Berenfeld O, Hocini M, et al. Spectral analysis identifies sites of high-frequency activity maintaining atrial fibrillation in humans. *Circulation* 2005;112:789–97.

Sanders P, Hocini M, Jais P, et al. Characterization of focal atrial tachycardia using high-density mapping. *J Am Coll Cardiol* 2005;46:2088–99.

Schauerte P, Scherlag BJ, Patterson E, et al. Focal atrial fibrillation: experimental evidence for a pathophysiologic role of the autonomic nervous system. *J Cardiovasc Electrophysiol* 2001;12:592–9.

Takahashi Y, Hocini M, O'Neill MD, et al. Sites of focal atrial activity characterized by endocardial mapping during atrial fibrillation. *J Am Coll Cardiol* 2006;47:2005–12.

Takahashi Y, O'Neill MD, Hocini M, et al. Effects of stepwise ablation of chronic atrial fibrillation on atrial electrical and mechanical properties. *J Am Coll Cardiol* 2007;49:1306–14.

Takahashi Y, O'Neill MD, Hocini M, et al. Characterization of electrograms associated with termination of chronic atrial fibrillation by catheter ablation. *J Am Coll Cardiol* 2008;51:1003–10.

Verma A, Kilicaslan F, Adams JR, et al. Extensive ablation during pulmonary vein antrum isolation has no adverse impact on left atrial function: an echocardiography and cine computed tomography analysis. *J Cardiovasc Electrophysiol* 2006;17:741–6.

Wijffels MC, Kirchhof CJ, Dorland R, et al. Atrial fibrillation begets atrial fibrillation. A study in awake chronically instrumented goats. *Circulation* 1995;92:1954–68.

Abbreviations

AF	atrial fibrillation		LPV	left pulmonary vein
AFCL	atrial fibrillation cycle length		LSPV	left superior pulmonary vein
Ant	anterior		LSVC	left superior vena cava
AP	anteroposterior		MA	mitral annulus
AT	atrial tachycardia		MV	mitral valve
ATCL	atrial tachycardia cycle length		p	proximal
CFAE	continuous fractionated atrial electrogram		Post	posterior
			PPI	post-pacing interval
CL	cycle length		PRd	distal pole recording
CS	coronary sinus		PRp	proximal pole recording
CSd	distal coronary sinus		PV	pulmonary vein
CSm	mid-portion of coronary sinus		PVI	pulmonary vein isolation
CSp	proximal coronary sinus		PVP	pulmonary vein potential
CT	computed tomography		RA	right atrium
CTI	cavotricuspid isthmus		RAA	right atrial appendage
d	distal		RAO	right anterior oblique
ECG	electrocardiogram		RF	radiofrequency energy
EGM	electrogram		RFd	radiofrequency energy distal
Inf LA	inferior left atrium		RFp	radiofrequency energy proximal
IVC	inferior vena cava		RIPV	right inferior pulmonary vein
LA	left atrium		RPV	right pulmonary vein
LAA	left atrial appendage		RSPV	right superior pulmonary vein
LAO	left anterior oblique		SVC	superior vena cava
LIPV	left inferior pulmonary vein		TEE	transesophageal echocardiogram
LMWH	low-molecular-weight heparin		TV	tricuspid valve

Index

Page numbers in **bold** refer to figures.